Mosby's

Oncology
Nursing
Certification
Review

Mosby's
Oncology Nursing Certification Review

Cynthia C. Chernecky, RN, PhD, AOCN
Associate Professor
School of Nursing
Department of Adult Health
Medical College of Georgia
Augusta, Georgia

Sue Schlesselman, RN, MSN, OCN
Assistant Professor
Department of Nursing
Augusta State University
Augusta, Georgia

St. Louis Baltimore Boston Carlsbad Chicago Minneapolis New York Philadelphia Portland
London Milan Sydney Tokyo Toronto

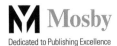

Editor-in-Chief: Sally Schrefer
Executive Editor: Barbara Nelson Cullen
Associate Developmental Editor: Eric Ham
Project Manager: John Rogers
Production Editor: Helen Hudlin
Designer: Kathi Gosche

FIRST EDITION
Copyright © 2000 by Mosby, Inc.

NOTICE

Pharmacology is an ever-changing field. Standard safety precautions must be followed, but as new research and clinical experience broaden our knowledge, changes in treatment and drug therapy may become necessary or appropriate. Readers are advised to check the most current product information provided by the manufacturer of each drug to be administered to verify the recommended dose, the method and duration of administration, and contraindications. It is the responsibility of the treating physician, relying on experience and knowledge of the patient, to determine dosages and the best treatment for each individual patient. Neither the Publisher nor the editor assume any liability for any injury and/or damage to persons or property arising from this publication.

The Publisher

Printed in the United States of America
Composition and Preparation by The Clarinda Company
Printing by Maple Vail Book Manufacturing Group

Mosby, Inc.
11830 Westline Industrial Drive
St. Louis, Missouri 63146

Internal Standard Book Number 0-323-00960-3

Library of Congress Cataloging-in-Publication Data
Chernecky, Cynthia C.
    Mosby's oncology nursing certification review / Cynthia Chernecky,
Sue Schlesselman. — 1st ed.
      p.   cm.
    Includes index.
    ISBN 0-323-00960-3
    1. Cancer—Nursing Examinations, questions, etc.
  I. Schlesselman, Sue. II. Title. III. Title: Oncology nursing
certification review.
    [DNLM: 1. Neoplasms—nursing Examination Questions. WY 18.2
C521m 2000]
RC266.C483 2000
610.73′698′076—dc21
DNLM/DLC
for Library of Congress   99-38245
                                    CIP

99 00 01 02 03 / 9 8 7 6 5 4 3 2 1

ACKNOWLEDGEMENTS

To those who make a difference in this world, and, particularly, unselfishly to my world. My heartfelt thanks to my mother Olga, late father Edward, Godmother Helen Prohorik, Goddaughter Priscilla, Godsons Jonathon and Vincent, brother Richard, nieces Ellie and Annie, nephew Michael, cousins Paula, Philip and Karyn, Mother Thecla and Mother Helena of Saints Mary and Martha Orthodox Monastery in South Carolina, His Eminence Archbishop DMITRI of the Orthodox Church in America, Father Gregory and Matuschka Raisa Koo, Father Peter and Matuschka Terri Smith, and Father David and Matuschka Sherri Garretson. A special acknowledgement to the universities that have added to my search for knowledge; the University of Connecticut, Yale University, University of Pittsburgh, Clemson University, Case Western Reserve University, the Medical College of Georgia, and the University of California-Los Angeles. And finally, to my co-editor Sue, and Barbara Nelson Cullen and Eric Ham at Mosby, Inc., and all persons within oncology nursing to whom I truly share a special place in my heart, I personally thank you.

CINDA CHERNECKY

I am grateful for those who provided a foundation for me as I ventured into new territory with this project. First and foremost, I am indebted to Cinda Chernecky who not only afforded me this opportunity, but sustained me with her endless encouragement, patience, and support. I have the utmost respect for Cinda, and I am in awe of her scholarly insight, positive attitude, and writing expertise.

A special thanks to Jean Balogh, a kindred spirit, who has been there in word and deed during my moments of trials and triumph. She is a constant source of motivation and strength.

I would like to extend my appreciation to my colleagues at the Department of Nursing at Augusta State University who endured this project with me. I am privileged to work with Jean Balogh, Cynthia King, Letha Lierman, Ginger Marshall, Charlotte Price, Sharon Vincent, and Melissa Williams, whose commitment to quality nursing education is unsurpassed.

My gratitude to those who support me as an oncology nurse and as a friend: Kim Bogart, Patti Butts, Bill and Kae Owen, Patty Lillis, Judi Peckel, and Sharon Vincent. Also, a sincere thanks to my parents, Merrill and Delores Schouten, who provide much encouragement and support via the telephone lines.

A special acknowledgement to Barbara Nelson Cullen and Eric Ham of Mosby for facilitating my participation in this project. And finally, I am grateful and humbled by the lives I have touched as an oncology nurse, but more important is the fact that all these individuals have touched me a thousandfold.

SUE SCHLESSELMAN

PREFACE

Knowledge is a source of strength, not just for one's self, but for those for whom we care. We have written this review book as a resource for our fellow nurse colleagues who, like ourselves, find reviews of basic and advanced oncology nursing a need and a comfort. This book corresponds to test taking for both the generalist and advanced oncology certification examinations and the chapter content features all areas of the Core Curriculm with a percentage of questions derived from the Oncology Nursing Certification Corporation's blueprint for the certification examination. Each chapter has multiple choice questions with a corresponding rationale to best enhance adult learning. Questions reflecting advanced oncology nursing content are indicated with an asterisk. We hope you find this book useful in your quest for general and advanced oncology nursing knowledge.

CONTENTS

Part VII: Health Promotion

Part VIII: Professional Performance

QUALITY OF LIFE

PART I

1

Comfort

QUESTIONS

1. Samantha had a thyroidectomy four months ago for treatment of medullary cancer of the thyroid. Even though she takes oxycodone with acetaminophen (Percocet), dysphagia still causes her to grimace. What type of pain is Samantha experiencing?
   a. Acute cancer pain.
   b. Chronic cancer pain.
   c. Acute noncancer pain.
   d. Chronic noncancer pain.

2. Which of the following is an example of somatic pain?
   a. Burning sensation in the abdominal region.
   b. Aching sensation in the right shoulder.
   c. Cramping sensation in the thigh region.
   d. Squeezing sensation to the lower back.

3. In teaching a patient about drug tolerance related to opioid pain medication, it is important to note that:
   a. It is the same phenomenon as addiction.
   b. It is a physiologic occurrence which the patient can control.
   c. Higher drug dosage will be needed to obtain a desired effect.
   d. Physical dependence is the same phenomenon.

4. Pain from bone metastases is most common in which type of cancer?
   a. Kidney.
   b. Colon.
   c. Bladder.
   d. Prostate.

5. An appropriate nonopioid analgesic to use for mild pain is:
   a. Ibuprofen (Advil).
   b. Oxycodone.
   c. Lorazepam (Ativan).
   d. Dipyridamole (Persantine).

6. A patient with breast cancer is experiencing moderate pain to her back and flank areas. The nurse expects the patient to be started on:
   a. Levorphanol tartate (Levo-Dromoran).
   b. Hydrocodone with acetaminophen (Vicodin).
   c. Fentanyl (Duragesic).
   d. Hydromorphone (Dilaudid).

7. A patient with ovarian cancer is experiencing bladder spasms. Which drug will best alleviate this symptom?
   a. Hydroxyzine (Vistaril).
   b. Alprazolam (Xanax).
   c. Belladonna and opium (B & O).
   d. Dexamethasone (Decadron).

8. Peripheral neuropathic pain is best treated with:
   a. Diazepam (Valium).
   b. Phenytoin (Dilantin).
   c. Indomethacin (Indocin).
   d. Fentanyl (Duragesic).

9. A patient with metastatic cancer reports continuous burning, lancinating pain to his legs and groin area despite being prescribed opioids and antidepressants. The patient should be started on which medication next?
  a. Haloperidol (Haldol).
  b. Ketorolac (Toradol).
  c. Lorazepam (Ativan).
  d. Cyclobenzaprine (Flexeril).

10. In treating elderly cancer patients with opioids, it is important to avoid a common misconception that:
  a. Pain is a normal part of aging.
  b. Advanced age results in prolonged half-lives of opioids.
  c. There is a higher risk of drug interactions.
  d. Lower initial doses of opioids may be needed.

11. Corticosteroids may be used to treat pain that is the result of:
  a. Organ obstruction.
  b. Muscle spasm.
  c. Neuropathic pain.
  d. Nerve compression.

12. A 4-year-old child with acute lymphoblastic leukemia has just undergone a lumbar puncture. The most appropriate method to assess the child's pain is to:
  a. Use the pain faces assessment tool.
  b. Ask the child to rate the pain from one to 10.
  c. Use the poker chip assessment tool.
  d. Ask the child's adult caregiver.

13. A patient taking haloperidol (Haldol) as an adjuvant treatment for pain is experiencing intermittent jerking of facial muscles and eye spasms. The nurse should treat these symptoms with:
  a. Dextroamphetamine (Dexedrine).
  b. Clonazepam (Klonopin).
  c. Diphenhydramine (Benadryl).
  d. Baclofen (Lioresal).

14. A patient with bone metastases who is prescribed a multidrug pain management regimen reports bruising and epigastric pain. The causative drug is most likely:
  a. Choline magnesium trisalicylate (Trilisate).
  b. Meperidine (Demerol).
  c. Nortriptyline (Pamelor).
  d. Naproxen (Naprosyn).

15. A patient has difficulties stating the intensity of her pain. The nurse suggests which of the following to assist with this problem?
  a. Ask the patient to report how the pain changes over time.
  b. Ask the patient to describe the pain in detail.
  c. Show the patient how to use a numerical scale to describe the pain.
  d. Instruct the patient to point to the pain location.

16. A patient reports to the nurse that he waits and takes his oral immediate-release morphine only when the pain is severe. It is important the patient understands that:
  a. Switching to oxycodone may provide better control.
  b. Pain medication taken before the pain gets severe is more effective.
  c. Severe pain is related to disease progression.
  d. Immediate-release morphine is the drug of choice with pain.

17. Mr. Jones has begun taking immediate-release oral morphine at a dosage of 30 mg every 4 to 6 hours for pain related to his colon cancer. The nurse teaches him to assess for which side effect?
    a. Urinary retention.
    b. Hypertension.
    c. Increased ventilatory volume.
    d. Insomnia.

18. The nurse is evaluating discharge education for a patient receiving long-acting analgesics for cancer pain. The nurse knows the patient has an understanding of the discharge instructions when the patient states:
    a. "I will make sure to take my pain medication at meals to minimize side effects."
    b. "I will take my medication at fixed intervals to get the best effect."
    c. "It's important I take this medication every four hours to obtain pain relief."
    d. "I can take the medication as needed and still receive pain control benefits."

19. An example of distraction to provide pain relief is:
    a. Biofeedback.
    b. Exercise.
    c. Music.
    d. Massage.

20. A patient with lung cancer is to begin a pain control regimen with morphine. The preferred initial route of analgesia is:
    a. Oral.
    b. Transdermal.
    c. Rectal.
    d. Subcutaneous.

21. Which of the following treatments does not usually cause fatigue?
    a. Granulocyte-macrophage colony-stimulating factor.
    b. Interleukin-2.
    c. Interferon.
    d. Tumor necrosis factor.

22. In assessing the timing, duration, and patterns of fatigue, the nurse is assessing which dimension of fatigue?
    a. Affective dimension.
    b. Behavioral dimension.
    c. Sensory dimension
    d. Temporal dimension.

23. A chemotherapy patient is experiencing fatigue-related anemia. The physician has ordered erythropoietin (Procrit). The nurse expects the patient to be prescribed a starting dose of:
    a. 100 U/kg SQ three times per week.
    b. 150 U/kg SQ three times per week.
    c. 300 U/kg SQ three times per week.
    d. 450 U/kg SQ three times per week.

24. Concentration is often impaired with fatigue. Which assessment method would best provide data regarding a patient's ability to concentrate?
    a. Have the patient describe any problems.
    b. Ask the patient to state date and time.
    c. Ask the patient to recall words given from a list.
    d. Perform an observational exam of the patient.

25. According to the Piper Fatigue Questionnaire, a patient given a "1" on the fatigue toxicity scale is experiencing:
    a. Mild fatigue.
    b. Moderate fatigue.
    c. Severe fatigue.
    d. Overwhelming fatigue.

26. What is an important intervention when using the Piper Fatigue Questionnaire?
    a. Consider the time of the day the questionnaire is completed.
    b. The questionnaire is to be completed by the patient.
    c. Another assessment tool may be needed since the questionnaire is not multidimensional.
    d. The questionnaire should always be used to gather information about fatigue.

27. A patient with breast cancer informs the nurse that on nights when she doesn't feel fatigued, she stays up to catch up on unfinished household tasks. The nurse's best response to this is:
    a. "It is important that you maintain a regular pattern of when you go to bed."
    b. "Your anxiety level is probably lowered after you accomplish those tasks."
    c. "You could ignore those tasks and concentrate on other aspects of your well being."
    d. "As long as you exercise during the day, a late bed time will not affect you very much."

28. A nurse is teaching a patient undergoing radiation therapy about exercises that can minimize fatigue. Which of the following should not be included in the teaching?
    a. Walking.
    b. Swimming.
    c. Aerobic exercises.
    d. Golf.

29. Which of the following malignancies has a high potential for causing pruritis?
    a. Squamous cell lung cancer.
    b. Multiple myeloma.
    c. Esophageal cancer.
    d. Basal cell carcinoma.

30. Which of the following laboratory findings are expected in a patient experiencing pruritis?
    a. Hypoglycemia.
    b. Hyperuricemia.
    c. Decreased blood urea nitrogen.
    d. Decreased serum creatinine.

31. Which of the following nursing diagnoses is most appropriate for a patient experiencing pruritis?
    a. Fluid volume deficit.
    b. Self-care deficit.
    c. Impaired tissue integrity.
    d. Fear.

32. A patient with pruritis should be taught to:
    a. Take warm baths twice a day.
    b. Keep room humidity at 40%.
    c. Eat a high-carbohydrate diet.
    d. Scratch areas of pruritis carefully.

33. Medication therapy to treat acral erythema may include the use of:
    a. Amitriptyline (Elavil).
    b. Acetaminophen (Tylenol).
    c. Pyridoxine (Doxine).
    d. Dipyridamole (Persantine).

34. A patient who received chemotherapy and radiation therapy for breast cancer has developed ulcerated sores under the breasts. The most appropriate nursing care would include:
    a. Apply antibiotic ointment to the area and cover with gauze.
    b. Apply wet-to-wet dressings every 8 hours.
    c. Use petroleum-based lotion on the area and cover with gauze.
    d. Take a shower twice daily to cleanse the ulcerated area.

35. A patient with recurrent sarcoma experiences a reddened area on his right arm 1 day after radiation. The nurse instructs the patient to do which of the following to treat radiation recall?
    a. Apply warm, wet compresses to the area.
    b. Take hydroxyzine (Vistaril) as needed.
    c. Apply cool, wet compresses to the area.
    d. Elevate the arm to the level of the heart.

36. A patient has a generalized macular, papular rash caused by aminoglutethimide (Cytadren). The patient is experiencing pruritis. Pharmacologic management of this skin disorder includes all of the following EXCEPT:
    a. Cholestyramine (Prevalite).
    b. Cimetidine (Tagamet).
    c. Diphenhydramine (Benadryl).
    d. Chlorpheniramine (Chlorate).

37. A natural product the nurse may suggest a patient use in the bath to soothe pruritis is:
    a. Glycerin.
    b. Beeswax.
    c. Oatmeal.
    d. Calamine.

38. A patient with stage IIIB Hodgkin's disease informs his nurse that he is having sleep disturbances. The nurse suspects a cause of the sleep disturbance may be:
    a. Xerostomia.
    b. Delerium.
    c. An electrolyte imbalance.
    d. Night sweats.

39. A patient is having difficulty falling asleep at night. With a tentative diagnosis of insomnia, the nurse can expect to find which of the following signs and symptoms?
    a. Focused thinking.
    b. Irritability.
    c. Improved concentration.
    d. Minimal daytime drowsiness.

40. The nurse is assessing Ms. Brooks, a newly hospitalized cancer patient. To collect objective data about the patient's sleep patterns the nurse should:
    a. Observe the patient for yawning and nystagmus.
    b. Ask the patient how many hours of sleep she gets nightly.
    c. Determine if the patient uses sleep aids.
    d. Ask the patient how much coffee and cola she drinks daily.

41. When teaching a patient about cognitive strategies to promote sleep, the nurse realizes more instruction is needed when the patient states the following:
    a. "I can count sheep to help me fall asleep."
    b. "Prayer every night will help me to relax."
    c. "A massage will help me to calm down."
    d. "Imagery of pleasant places may help me to go to sleep easier."

*42. Mr. Tate is a 65-year-old patient with lung cancer who completed a second cycle of chemotherapy 10 days ago. He has altered peripheral circulation secondary to diabetes mellitus. He is now complaining of burning-type pain to his flank areas. The nurse suspects the patient is experiencing:
    a. Peripheral neuropathy.
    b. Phantom pain.
    c. Herpetic neuralgia.
    d. Psychogenic pain.

*43. A patient receiving morphine (Duramorph) through an epidural catheter is experiencing pruritis. Which of the following agents should be used to alleviate the pruritis?
    a. Nalbuphine (Nubain).
    b. Nalmefene hydrochloride (Revex).
    c. Nefazodone (Serzone).
    d. Naloxone (Narcan).

*44. On a follow-up visit, a patient with pancreatic cancer reports difficulties in falling asleep and staying asleep. Physical examination reveals hypertension, weight loss, and muscle weakness. The nurse suspects the patient has developed which paraneoplastic syndrome?
    a. Paraneoplastic erythrocytosis.
    b. Syndrome of inappropriate antidiuresis.
    c. Hypercalcemia-associated syndrome.
    d. Adrenocorticotropic hormone syndrome.

*45. Mrs. Shelley is a 48-year-old woman with colon cancer. She calls the oncology nurse to report crampy, abdominal pain. She also is experiencing the need to urinate hourly. Her medications include 60 mg of slow-release morphine three times per day, 10 mg of prochlorperazine (Compazine) every 6 hours for nausea, and 25 mg amitriptyline (Elavil) at bedtime for sleep. A suspected cause of the patient's symptom is:
    a. Patient noncompliance with the medical regimen.
    b. Metastatic disease to the bone.
    c. Side effects of her medications.
    d. Nerve compression causing a plexopathetic syndrome.

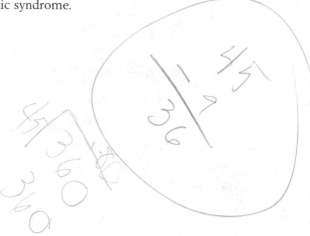

* Reflects advanced oncology nursing content

Answers

1. **(a)** The patient is experiencing acute cancer pain because the pain is related to the treatment for her cancer. Also, the location of the pain is known, objective pain behaviors are exhibited, and the pain has lasted less than 6 months.

2. **(b)** Somatic pain is characterized by aching or gnawing sensations in a well-localized area of the body.

3. **(c)** After repetitive doses of opioid medications, the dosage loses its effectiveness, thus requiring higher doses to achieve pain control. This phenomenon is known as drug tolerance.

4. **(d)** Prostate cancer has a high incidence of metastases to the bone.

5. **(a)** Ibuprofen is an appropriate choice for mild pain.

6. **(b)** Moderate cancer pain should be treated with a weak opioid with or without an adjuvant. Hydrocodone with acetaminophen (Vicodin) is a weak opioid with an adjuvant.

7. **(c)** Belladonna and opium soothes gastrointestinal and bladder spasms.

8. **(b)** Anticonvulsants such as phenytoin (Dilantin) provide relief from peripheral neuropathic pain.

9. **(a)** Haloperidol (Haldol) may be prescribed to treat continuous neuropathic pain.

10. **(a)** Pain is not a normal aspect of growing older.

11. **(d)** Corticosteroids are used to relieve pain associated with nerve compression.

12. **(a)** The pain faces assessment tool is appropriate for a 4-year-old child to use to report his or her pain.

13. **(c)** Diphenhydramine (Benadryl) is treatment for extrapyramidal effects.

14. **(d)** Naproxen can inhibit platelet aggregation, thus leading to gastritis or bleeding tendencies.

15. **(c)** Intensity of pain is best described using a numerical scale.

16. **(b)** Pain medication should be taken before the pain is severe for optimal results to be achieved.

17. **(a)** Urinary retention is an adverse effect of opioid analgesics.

18. **(b)** Long-acting analgesics should be scheduled at fixed intervals to achieve a sustained and balanced effect.

19. **(c)** Music serves as a distraction to provide relief of pain.

20. **(a)** The oral route is convenient and is usually less expensive than other routes.

21. **(a)** Granulocyte-macrophage colony-stimulating factor is not a usual cause of fatigue.

22. **(d)** Temporal dimension is related to data about timing and patterns of fatigue.

23. **(b)** A starting dose of erythropoietin (Procrit) is 150 U/kg three times per week.

24. **(c)** A patient's ability to concentrate can be tested by having the patient recall words from a list.

25. **(a)** Using the fatigue toxicity scale from the Piper Fatigue Questionnaire, a rating of "1" indicates mild fatigue.

26. **(a)** An important intervention when using the Piper Fatigue Questionnaire is to administer it when a patient feels less fatigued. Generally, less fatigue is experienced in the morning hours.

27. **(a)** Going to bed at a regular time minimizes fatigue by maintaining circadian rhythms.

28. **(c)** Aerobic exercises may actually increase a sense of fatigue.

29. **(b)** Multiple myeloma is associated with causing pruritis.

30. **(b)** Hyperuricemia may be present in a patient experiencing pruritis.

31. **(c)** An appropriate nursing diagnosis is impaired tissue integrity related to the itching and scratching accompanying pruritis.

32. **(b)** Room humidity of 40% decreases moisture loss from the skin.

33. **(c)** Pyridoxine, 50 mg TID, may be ordered to treat acral erythema.

34. **(a)** For ulceration or erosions that occur from radiation, the involved area should receive an application of antibiotic ointment and then be covered with a gauze dressing.

35. **(c)** The application of cool, wet compresses promotes vasoconstriction and soothes the affected area.

36. **(a)** Cholestyramine (Prevalite) is used to treat pruritis; however, it is effective only when the pruritis is caused by elevated levels of bile salts.

37. **(c)** Oatmeal added to a bath can soothe pruritis.

38. **(d)** Night sweats from Hodgkin's disease often disturb sleep.

39. **(b)** An individual with insomnia is likely to experience irritability.

40. **(a)** Observation is a method to collect objective data. The other methods are subjective.

41. **(c)** A massage may be useful in helping a person fall asleep, but it is not considered a cognitive strategy.

*42. **(c)** The immune suppressive effects of chemotherapy increase a patient's risk for activation of the varicella-zoster virus. Symptoms of varicella-zoster infections include burning, aching, and lancinating-type pain occurring along the distribution of nerves, often in the flank or trunk.

* Reflects advanced oncology nursing content

*43. **(a)** Pruritis caused by intraspinal infusion of opioids should be treated with an agonist-antagonist agent.

*44. **(d)** Increased endogenous corticosteroid production, as with adrenocorticotropic hormone syndrome, causes sleep disorders as well as muscle weakness, weight loss, and hypertension.

*45. **(c)** The combined anticholinergic side effects of the patient's medication regimen are causing symptoms of urinary retention.

* Reflects advanced oncology nursing content

2

Coping: Psychosocial Issues

QUESTIONS

1. A 36-year-old woman has just received a diagnosis of stage II cervical cancer. Situational factors that may affect her emotional distress regarding the cancer diagnosis include all of the following EXCEPT:
   a. Role responsibilities.
   b. Personality traits.
   c. Social support.
   d. Family communication.

2. Emotional distress in a cancer patient differs from anxiety in that:
   a. Feelings are related to specific stressors regarding cancer.
   b. The duration of the emotionally distressing thoughts lasts longer.
   c. The presence of nervousness and worry are more intense.
   d. The presence of physical symptoms generally does not occur.

3. The night before a scheduled mastectomy, a hospitalized patient is having trouble sleeping despite using a hypnotic medication. The patient asks the nurse to sit with her for awhile. What is the nurse's most appropriate response?
   a. "I realize the hospital is not a place to get much rest, but what else can I do to make you more comfortable so you can sleep?"
   b. "You seem to have insomnia. It's important for you to sleep, so I will see about giving you some more sleep medication."
   c. "I imagine you're worried about your procedure tomorrow. The procedure you will be undergoing is quite routine and your recovery should be quite unremarkable."
   d. "You seem to have your mind on something. Do you have concerns or questions about something?"

4. General medical interventions to treat emotional distress include all of the following EXCEPT:
   a. Individual counseling.
   b. Spiritual counseling.
   c. Guided imagery.
   d. Hypnotic medication.

5. A patient presents to the emergency room stating "my chest feels heavy and it's hard for me to breathe. I suppose it's because of the lung cancer the doctor found 2 days ago." Physical examination reveals tachypnea, diaphoresis, irregular heartbeat, elevated blood pressure, and restlessness. After the physician rules out any physical cause for the symptoms, the nurse assigns the following nursing diagnosis to the patient:
   a. Disturbed self-esteem related to diagnosis of terminal illness.
   b. Altered role performance related to diagnosis of cancer.
   c. Fear related to diagnosis of terminal illness.
   d. Anxiety related to recent diagnosis of cancer.

6. During infusion of chemotherapy, a patient begins to cry, attempts to pull the intravenous line out, and tries to get up out of her chair. The first nursing action is to:
   a. Stay physically close to the patient.
   b. Tell the patient to calm down.
   c. Ask the patient to verbalize her fears.
   d. Divert the patient's attention.

7. Which of the following statements reflects the patient's understanding of minimizing anxiety?
   a. "It is helpful to think about my uneasy feelings in order to deal with the anxiety."
   b. "I will only drink two cups of coffee a day."
   c. "Since I don't know why I have these feelings, there's no need to identify the causes."
   d. "Smoking will help me feel better."

8. In assessing for severe anxiety reactions, the nurse should monitor for:
   a. Panic attacks.
   b. Catatonia.
   c. Seizures.
   d. Ataxia.

9. A patient reports drowsiness since starting therapy with an anti-anxiety medication. To minimize drowsiness the nurse suggests to:
   a. Decrease the amount of daily protein in the diet.
   b. Exercise twice daily.
   c. Increase intake of iced tea and cola.
   d. Take the scheduled dose at bedtime.

10. Assessment findings that may indicate depression include:
   a. Slowed speech, lack of eye contact, crying.
   b. Labile emotions, hyperventilation, hand tremors.
   c. Slowed speech, disorientation, minimal eye contact.
   d. Hyperventilation, diaphoresis, unkempt appearance.

11. A highly effective intervention in working with a patient with depression is:
   a. Initiating symptom management.
   b. Providing disease information.
   c. Listening unconditionally.
   d. Validating thoughts.

12. Even though a patient was informed that blurred vision could be a side effect from his antidepressant therapy, he asks the nurse how to deal with it. The nurse's best response is:
   a. "You may want to consider purchasing eyeglasses to correct the problem."
   b. "You will experience less blurred vision as time goes on, so continue with your therapy."
   c. "Rest your eyes during the day by taking several short naps."
   d. "Continue your usual routine and you'll notice you're distracted from the blurred vision."

13. For a hospitalized cancer patient, which of the following is *not* a treatment-related barrier to practicing spiritual rituals?
   a. Confinement in isolation room.
   b. Dietary restriction.
   c. Lack of privacy.
   d. Embarrassment related to spiritual practices.

14. Which of the following is a serious consequence of a cancer patient experiencing spiritual distress?
   a. Loneliness.
   b. Noncompliance with a prescribed medical regimen.
   c. Personal conflict.
   d. Social isolation.

15. Nursing interventions appropriate for the patient experiencing spiritual distress include:
    a. Discussing personal values with the patient regarding spirituality.
    b. Stressing the importance of faith in the prescribed therapeutic regimen.
    c. Contacting the patient's spiritual support person to meet with the patient.
    d. Assuring the patient that therapy will not interfere with the patient's spiritual practices.

16. The nurse suspects a patient is feeling spiritual distress when the patient asks which of the following questions?
    a. "Why do I have to suffer with cancer?"
    b. "How do the nurses work with cancer patients all the time?"
    c. "I feel I will be stronger after going through cancer treatment."
    d. "Will the chaplain come visit while I'm here?"

17. Loss of personal control may be caused by which of the following disease-related factors?
    a. Ineffective interpersonal relations.
    b. Debilitating, progressive symptoms.
    c. Ambiguous decision making.
    d. Altered personal space.

18. A patient with bladder cancer states to the nurse, "I don't even know why I continue to watch my diet and take my medicine, because the cancer is going to do what it wants to do." The nurse recognizes the patient is experiencing:
    a. Aggression.
    b. Powerlessness.
    c. Anxiety.
    d. Depression.

19. Which of the following would be an appropriate outcome statement for a patient experiencing loss of personal control?
    a. Has healthy and satisfying interpersonal relationship.
    b. Achieves motivation in providing self-care.
    c. States methods to get involved with cancer treatment.
    d. Understands complications that can occur from loss of control.

20. To plan effective interventions to minimize a patient's sense of loss of control, the nurse asks which of the following questions?
    a. "Are you satisfied with your involvement in your plan of care?"
    b. "How are you feeling?"
    c. "What aspect of your health care would you like to talk about?"
    d. "Are you receiving support from others?"

21. Grief may be defined as the emotional response to:
    a. The change in lifestyle related to aging.
    b. The death of a family member or friend.
    c. An illness with a poor prognosis.
    d. The loss of a valued person or possession.

22. Which of the following is considered to be a dysfunctional grief response?
    a. A 64-year-old widow of 2 years who "sees" her dead husband in public crowds when she is out in public.
    b. A 48-year-old widow of 8 months who cries easily at the mention of her dead husband's name.
    c. The husband of a 36-year-old breast cancer patient tells the hospice nurse, "I am ready for her to die."
    d. A 70-year-old widow of 6 months who reports hearing his dead wife's voice at night when he is in bed.

23. While working with a dying patient's family, the patient's son states, "If mom would get better I promise to be a better son." The nurse realizes the son is experiencing which characteristic of the loss and grief process?
    a. Shock.
    b. Acute mourning.
    c. Restitution.
    d. Acceptance.

24. Which of the following is a psychological reaction to loss and grief?
    a. Loss of appetite.
    b. Decreased levels of energy.
    c. Disturbed sleep pattern.
    d. Inability to concentrate.

25. Strategies to facilitate coping with the grief response include all of the following EXCEPT:
    a. Assisting to identify personal strengths.
    b. Teaching relaxation techniques.
    c. Providing instruction regarding sedative medications.
    d. Referring to a support group.

26. Mrs. Locke was just admitted to the surgical unit after undergoing a bilateral mastectomy. To address the patient's sense of loss, it is important for the nurse to initially:
    a. Validate the patient's grief reaction.
    b. Monitor the patient for hostility.
    c. Not address the issue of loss.
    d. Call a representative from Reach to Recovery.

27. After speaking with a woman about the death of her husband 8 weeks ago, the nurse is concerned the woman is becoming withdrawn. Which nursing diagnosis most accurately describes this complication of grief?
    a. Denial.
    b. Social isolation.
    c. Sleep pattern disturbance.
    d. Low self-esteem.

28. A hospice nurse caring for a homebound patient notices that the spouse is starting to distance herself from the patient. The nurse suspects that the spouse is experiencing:
    a. Resolved grief.
    b. Dysfunctional grief.
    c. Disenfranchised grief.
    d. Anticipatory grief.

29. Which of the following interventions is least helpful in assisting an individual to adapt to the reactions of grief?
    a. Provide anticipatory guidance.
    b. Encourage open communication.
    c. Refer to counseling.
    d. Advocate for the expression of only positive feelings.

30. A colon cancer patient who continually phones in sick to work even though his disease is under control is exhibiting:
    a. Social dysfunction.
    b. Hopelessness.
    c. Apathy.
    d. Social separation.

31. All of the following are cancer disease–related factors that can influence social dysfunction EXCEPT:
    a. Unpleasant side effects.
    b. Body structure changes.
    c. Substance abuse.
    d. Inadequate symptom control.

32. To minimize dysfunctional behavior for a sarcoma patient who underwent left arm amputation, the nurse should refer the patient to:
    a. Occupational therapy.
    b. Psychotherapy.
    c. Social counseling.
    d. Pastoral care.

33. Patient behavior that may indicate social dysfunction is:
    a. Self-blame.
    b. Blaming others for personal problems.
    c. Irritability.
    d. Self-doubt.

34. When assessing family resources in regard to social functioning, the nurse should obtain important information regarding the makeup of the family group as well as the:
    a. Educational levels of the family members.
    b. Cleanliness of the family residence.
    c. Quality of the family relationships.
    d. Belief systems of the family members.

35. A patient with metatastic kidney cancer is now bed bound after experiencing compression of the spinal cord. In preparation for the patient's discharge to home, the nurse needs to assess for which of the following?
    a. The family's ability and willingness to care for the patient.
    b. The family's willingness to use community resources.
    c. The patient's ability to verbalize needs.
    d. The patient's understanding of compliance with a medical regimen.

*36. Mrs. Potter has emotional distress associated with a recent diagnosis of stage III ovarian cancer. Her distress has negatively affected her lifestyle and physical well-being. She is at high risk for the development of which major psychiatric disorder?
   a. Depression.
   b. Anorexia nervosa.
   c. Schizophrenia.
   d. Self-esteem disturbance.

*37. A patient has a history of chronic anxiety disorder associated with panic attacks. The doctor has noted in the progress notes that the patient now has a psychosomatic illness. Which of the following is a psychosomatic illness?
   a. Shortness of breath.
   b. Vertigo.
   c. Menstrual irregularities.
   d. Migraine headaches.

*38. A 58-year-old man with lung cancer is brought to the clinic by his wife. She reports a rapid onset of confusion, irritability, hypersomnia, and recurrent talk of death. The clinic nurse suspects the patient is experiencing:
   a. Drug withdrawal.
   b. Delirium.
   c. Depression.
   d. Dementia.

*39. A patient with head and neck cancer has been hospitalized for intractable nausea and vomiting. The patient smokes two packs of cigarettes per day and has a history of alcohol abuse. He becomes verbally abusive in stating his anger about potentially losing his job as a result of being hospitalized. The nurse is aware that the patient is showing characteristics of:
   a. Loss of control.
   b. Delusional behavior.
   c. Social dysfunction.
   d. Schizoaffective disorder.

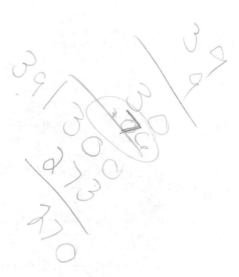

ANSWERS

1. **(b)**   Personality traits are developmental factors that affect emotional distress.

2. **(a)**   Unlike anxiety, emotional distress has a specific stress or stressor related to cancer, which can be identified.

3. **(d)**   Responding by acknowledging a problem and following with an open-ended question may allow a patient to ventilate thoughts, fears, and concerns about an issue or situation.

4. **(d)**   Hypnotics are used less frequently to treat emotional distress. Sedatives, anxiolytics, and antidepressants are usually used.

5. **(d)**   The patient is exhibiting signs and symptoms of anxiety. The patient may be experiencing anxiety related to a new cancer diagnosis.

6. **(a)**   Staying physically close to the patient provides for initial safety, and it demonstrates the nurse is present to support the patient.

7. **(b)**   Limiting or omitting alcohol, caffeine, and nicotine assists in minimizing anxiety and symptoms of anxiety.

8. **(a)**   Panic attacks are a reaction to severe anxiety.

9. **(d)**   Taking the scheduled dose of anti-anxiety medication at bedtime may decrease daytime drowsiness.

10. **(a)**   Physical findings of depression include slowed speech, lack of eye contact, and crying.

11. **(c)**   Active listening in a supportive environment promotes a trusting nurse-patient relationship.

12. **(b)**   Compliance with the antidepressant therapy is important, so reassurance that blurred vision may diminish is important to communicate to the patient.

13. **(d)**   Embarrassment over spiritual practices is a situational factor that may cause spiritual distress in a cancer patient.

14. **(b)**   Noncompliance with a prescribed medical regimen is a serious consequence of spiritual distress.

15. **(c)**   Contacting the patient's spiritual resource person assists to support the patient's spiritual beliefs.

16. **(a)**   The patient is questioning the meaning of suffering, which can be a defining characteristic for spiritual distress.

17. **(b)**   Debilitating, progressive symptoms are disease-related factors that contribute to loss of personal control.

18. **(b)**   Apathy and feelings of resignation are common characteristics of loss of personal control.

19. **(c)**   This outcome is measurable and provides a way for a patient to get involved, thus minimizing loss of personal control.

20. **(a)**   Allowing the patient to report on the amount of involvement with a plan of care helps to assess for loss of personal control. Involvement provides a sense of control.

21. **(d)**   The most encompassing definition of grief is the loss of a valued person or possession.

22. **(a)**   Two years after the death of a significant other, the surviving individual should rarely encounter "seeing" the image of the deceased in public places.

23. **(c)**   Restitution and bargaining are characteristics of the loss and grief process in which an individual attempts to change the outcome of the situation by promising to change personal behavior.

24. **(d)**   Inability to concentrate is one type of psychological reaction to loss and grief.

25. **(c)**   Sedating drugs are not useful in facilitating coping with the grief response.

26. **(a)**   Since the patient has experienced a loss, it is important to validate that the grief response is acceptable.

27. **(b)**   Social isolation can block the grief resolution process, causing complications to the coping process.

28. **(d)**   Anticipatory grief is the process of experiencing feelings of loss or emotional distance before the actual loss occurs.

29. **(d)**   Encouraging the expression of only positive feelings does not allow for full adaptation to grief, since negative feelings such as anger are also a part of grief.

30. **(a)**   Social dysfunction is defined as the inability to interact effectively with the environment, including one's community, occupational, and family environment.

31. **(c)**   Substance abuse is a general situational factor that can affect social dysfunction.

32. **(a)**   Occupational therapy facilitates the patient's adaptation to his amputation and allows the patient to interact in a functional manner.

33. **(b)**   Blaming others for personal problems is behavior that indicates not taking responsibility for one's actions, which can lead to social dysfunction.

34. **(c)**   The quality of family relationships is an important parameter to assess in relation to social functioning.

35. **(a)**   A family's willingness and ability to care for an ill family member is important to assess, because social dysfunction can occur with caregiver role strain.

*36. **(a)**   The patient is at risk for the development of anxiety or depression, with the risk of suicidal behavior.

*37. **(d)**   Migraine headaches can be considered a psychosomatic illness. Other psychosomatic illnesses include colitis and gastric ulcers.

*38. **(b)**   The acute onset of the symptoms of impaired cognitive function is indicative of delirium.

*39. **(c)**   Characteristics of social dysfunction include substance abuse, aggression, employment problems, legal difficulties, violence, and superficial relationships.

* Reflects advanced oncology nursing content

CHAPTER **3**

Coping: Altered Body Image and Alopecia

QUESTIONS

1. A serious risk of disturbed body image may be:
   a. Suicide.
   b. Loneliness.
   c. Anxiety.
   d. Loss of control.

2. A nurse develops outcomes to assist a young female patient in dealing with an above-the-knee amputation. Which outcome best addresses the issue of body image?
   a. Discusses ways her body structure has changed.
   b. Identifies methods to adapt to her previous job.
   c. States care of the amputation stump.
   d. Lists exercises she can do in physical therapy.

3. A patient's refusal to look at her mastectomy incision 10 days after the surgery may indicate a body image disturbance within which assessment area?
   a. Sexual.
   b. Physical.
   c. Cognitive.
   d. Psychosocial.

4. A female bone marrow transplant patient has experienced hyperpigmentation from her treatment. The best referral the nurse can make is to:
   a. Reach to Recovery.
   b. Can Surmount.
   c. Look Good, Feel Better.
   d. Candlelighters.

5. A male patient with a brain tumor is scheduled to receive standard radiation treatment totaling 50 Gy. In teaching about alopecia, it is important the nurse informs the patient that:
   a. Hair loss will be permanent.
   b. Scalp hypothermia can reduce hair loss.
   c. Hair loss will be temporary.
   d. Hair loss will be minimal.

6. An increased risk of infection exists when loss of hair is experienced from the:
   a. Scalp.
   b. Nares.
   c. Eyebrows.
   d. Pubic area.

7. Anticipatory teaching related to alopecia for a patient undergoing doxorubicin (Adriamycin) therapy should include telling the patient:
   a. Wash the hair and scalp frequently with a mild shampoo.
   b. Hair loss occurs over a period of weeks to months.
   c. Wigs or hairpieces should be obtained after hair loss occurs.
   d. Hair regrowth tends to start 6 to 8 weeks after completion of treatment.

8. Which of the following treatments is most likely to cause hair loss?
   a. Paclitaxel (Taxol).
   b. Thiotepa (Thioplex).
   c. Cytarabine (Cytosar-U).
   d. Vinorelbine (Navelbine).

*9. Six weeks ago a patient underwent radical cystectomy with placement of an ileal conduit. In the past week, the patient has experienced difficulty concentrating, indecisiveness, and avoidance of social interaction. Which of the following agents is recommended for this patient?
   a. Chlorpromazine (Thorazine).
   b. Haloperidol (Haldol).
   c. Lorazepam (Ativan).
   d. Gabapentin (Neurontin).

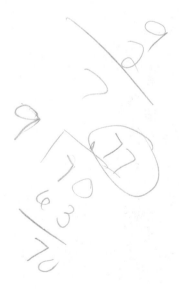

Answers

1. **(a)**   Suicide is a serious risk for a patient who is not able to adapt to changes in body image.

2. **(b)**   The identification of ways to reintegrate into previous roles is an appropriate outcome to help a patient deal with body image issues.

3. **(d)**   The refusal to look at a mastectomy incision, even several days after surgery, indicates a body image disturbance related to psychosocial issues.

4. **(c)**   Look Good, Feel Better is an organization to assist patients in skin care, hair care, and makeup.

5. **(a)**   When receiving radiation of over 40 Gy to an area, hair loss is permanent.

6. **(b)**   Loss of nasal hair decreases the body's normal line of defenses, thus increasing the risk for infection.

7. **(d)**   Hair regrowth tends to start 6 to 8 weeks after the completion of cancer treatment.

8. **(a)**   Paclitaxel (Taxol) has a high affinity for causing alopecia.

*9. **(c)**   Since the patient seems to be experiencing acute symptoms of anxiety, possibly related to body image alterations, a recommended treatment is lorazepam (Ativan).

---

* Reflects advanced oncology nursing content

4

Cultural Issues

QUESTIONS

1. The use of one's own culture as the method to judge others is termed:
   a. Ethnocentrism.
   b. Culture identity.
   c. Ethnic identity.
   d. Overgeneralization.

2. The highest overall cancer incidence rates occur among:
   a. Hispanic Americans.
   b. African Americans.
   c. Native Americans.
   d. Asian Americans.

3. Hispanics have the highest mortality rate for which of the following cancers?
   a. Cervical.
   b. Lung.
   c. Pancreas.
   d. Gallbladder.

4. Asian-Pacific Islanders are:
   a. The slowest-growing ethnic group in the U.S.
   b. The fastest-growing ethnic group in the U.S.
   c. Mostly from Japanese heritage.
   d. Mostly from Chinese heritage.

5. Which site is a leader in cancer incidence in the Japanese?
   a. Stomach.
   b. Breast.
   c. Lung.
   d. Brain.

6. Which of the following cancers occurs most frequently in Chinese Americans?
   a. Mouth and tongue cancer.
   b. Esophageal cancer.
   c. Nasopharyngeal cancer.
   d. Laryngeal cancer.

7. Among racial and ethnic groups, which group has the lowest 5-year survival rate from cancer?
   a. Mexican American.
   b. Native American.
   c. African American.
   d. Native Hawaiian.

8. Filipino women have the highest incidence rate for which cancer?
   a. Kidney.
   b. Breast.
   c. Cervical.
   d. Thyroid.

9. Which one of the following groups has the highest incidence and mortality rates for prostate cancer?
   a. African Americans.
   b. Hispanic Americans.
   c. Chinese Americans.
   d. Japanese Americans.

10. According to statistics from the American Cancer Society, which ethnic group has the highest 5-year cancer survival rate for all sites of cancer?
    a. Caucasian.
    b. Japanese.
    c. Chinese.
    d. Filipino.

11. Which of the following interventions is recommended when communicating with patients from another culture?
    a. Use casual language.
    b. Choose simple words.
    c. Pronounce the words louder.
    d. Focus on tasks rather than words.

12. Delayed screening and treatment of cancer may result from all of the following EXCEPT:
    a. Inability to pay for service.
    b. Limited access to health care.
    c. A sense of looking to the future.
    d. Lack of insurance.

13. During a teaching session a newly diagnosed cancer patient tells the nurse that his disease was caused by evil spirits from his ancestors. The nurse knows the patient has which type of health belief?
    a. Natural.
    b. Holistic.
    c. Biomedical.
    d. Magico-religious.

14. A nurse caring for a Hispanic American patient needs to be aware that an important component of therapy may involve a traditional healer known as a/an:
    a. Curandero.
    b. Herbalist.
    c. Root worker.
    d. Espirit.

15. An Asian woman just received a diagnosis of breast cancer. She appears distressed and withdrawn. The most appropriate nursing intervention is to:
    a. Touch her hand and ask her if she needs to talk about her situation.
    b. Ask her if she would like to discuss any of her concerns or fears.
    c. Sit and provide a silent presence to show support.
    d. Sit next to the patient, take her hand, and provide a silent presence to show support.

16. When assessing for biological variations in cultural groups, the nurse is aware that all of the following ethnic groups have lactose intolerance as a common problem EXCEPT:
    a. Hispanics.
    b. Native Americans.
    c. African Americans.
    d. Asians.

17. In regard to time orientation, which ethnic group values the future over the present?
    a. Asian.
    b. African.
    c. European.
    d. Hispanic.

18. Which of the following factors does not provide consistency in maintaining an individual's cultural heritage?
    a. Contact is maintained with an extended family.
    b. Ethnic customs are practiced.
    c. Education takes place in public schools.
    d. Family residences are located within an ethnic community.

19. When interviewing a Korean patient for a hospital admission, the patient provides only brief answers. The patient speaks quietly and appears unemotional. The nurse is aware that:
    a. This may be the normal communication pattern for the patient.
    b. The patient's behavior is suggestive of depression.
    c. A language barrier probably is present.
    d. Use of touch would facilitate the communication of the patient.

20. The main reason a nurse needs to obtain knowledge about culturally oriented care is to:
    a. Ensure each patient is treated equally.
    b. Integrate the patient's beliefs into the plan of care.
    c. Demonstrate to the patient that the nurse has knowledge of cultural differences.
    d. Provide individualized care that facilitates optimal functioning.

21. Accurately assessing a patient in terms of culture begins with:
    a. An awareness of the nurse's own culture.
    b. Sensitivity training to accept the uniqueness of others.
    c. Knowledge about various health practices of cultural groups.
    d. Adopting a philosophy of providing culturally competent care.

22. The social organization of a patient's cultural group is important to assess. Which of the following questions would NOT be helpful in determining the social organization of a cultural group?
    a. How is health defined?
    b. Is there a religious affiliation linked to the cultural group?
    c. Who is important in the decision-making process?
    d. What are the patient's roles?

23. The nurse is caring for a patient who only speaks Chinese. The nurse does not speak Chinese. When selecting an interpreter, it's important to choose a:
    a. Family member of the patient.
    b. Friend of the patient.
    c. Younger interpreter.
    d. Professional interpreter.

24. Vietnamese have the highest incidence for which of the following cancers?
    a. Oral cavity.
    b. Lung.
    c. Colon.
    d. Cervix.

25. Native Americans have high rates of disease associated with all of the following EXCEPT:
    a. Obesity.
    b. Alcohol.
    c. Tobacco.
    d. Illicit drugs.

*26. When caring for a patient of Asian descent, it is important to consider which of the following principles?
    a. Use touch often when communicating.
    b. The patient will often make decisions independently.
    c. Verbal expression is common when lack of understanding occurs.
    d. Keep time schedules flexible for the patient.

*27. While providing care to a Jamaican woman in her home a root worker arrives. The root worker administers herbs and elixirs to the patient that were not prescribed by the physician. The most appropriate nursing action is to:
    a. Analyze the types of herbs given to the patient.
    b. Explain to the patient the herbs were not prescribed by the doctor so they should not be used.
    c. Accept the patient's cultural right to use various modes of healing.
    d. Inform the patient of the advantages of her current therapies.

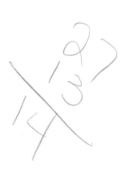

ANSWERS

1. **(a)**   Ethnocentrism is when others are viewed and judged according to one's own customs and culture.

2. **(b)**   When compared with other racial and ethnic groups, African Americans have the highest incidence rate of cancer in all sites.

3. **(d)**   Hispanic persons have the highest mortality rates for cancer of the gallbladder.

4. **(b)**   Asian-Pacific Islanders are the fastest growing ethnic group in the United States.

5. **(a)**   Stomach cancer is a leader in incidence among Japanese persons.

6. **(c)**   Nasopharyngeal cancer occurs most frequently in Chinese Americans.

7. **(b)**   Native Americans have the lowest 5-year survival rate from cancer.

8. **(d)**   Filipino women have the highest incidence rates for thyroid cancer.

9. **(a)**   African Americans have the highest incidence and mortality rates for prostate cancer.

10. **(b)**   Japanese persons have the highest 5-year survival rate for all sites of cancer.

11. **(b)**   The use of simple words spoken in the correct context and in a normal tone are recommended when trying to communicate with a patient from another culture.

12. **(c)**   Delayed screening and treatment is related to a focus on the present rather than the future.

13. **(d)**   Magico-religious health beliefs are based on the view that health and illness are influenced by supernatural forces.

14. **(a)**   A curandero is a traditional folk healer in the Hispanic culture.

15. **(c)**   The Asian culture generally prefers personal space not to be invaded, touch to be used rarely, and silence used as a method of communication.

16. **(b)**   Lactose intolerance is not a usual biological variation in Native Americans.

17. **(c)**   European ethnic groups tend to value the future over the present.

18. **(c)**   Education in public schools does not facilitate full ethnic or religious philosophies to be learned and practiced.

19. **(a)**   A patient of Korean ethnicity values silence, nonverbal communication, and the presence of family.

20. **(d)**   Individualized care is the primary reason nurses need to be aware and knowledgeable about cultural aspects of health care.

21. **(a)**   Awareness of one's own culture and its influences on one's behaviors and values is important in order to accurately assess patients within a cultural context. The understanding of one's own cultural perspective facilitates respect for the unfamiliar when working with patients from a different culture.

22. **(a)**   The cultural definition of health is an assessment parameter for learning about a patient's control within the environment.

23. **(d)**   A professional interpreter is the most appropriate choice.

24. **(d)**   Vietnamese people have the highest incidence of cervical cancer.

25. **(d)**   Illicit drug use is not a risk behavior highly associated with disease in Native Americans.

*26. **(d)**   The Asian culture generally values time in the present, thus time has a flexible characteristic. An Asian patient may arrive late for appointments because a strict schedule does not fit the value of time orientation in the present.

*27. **(c)**   Acceptance of the patient's right to use various modes of healing is important in providing culturally competent care. If traditional medicine is a valued part of the patient's culture, use of traditional medicine will occur in the midst of other treatment modalities.

* Reflects advanced oncology nursing content

5

Coping: Survivorship Issues and Financial Concerns

QUESTIONS

1. The most accurate definition of a cancer survivor is:
   a. An individual free of disease 5 years after a cancer diagnosis.
   b. A person diagnosed with cancer who experiences various processes along the cancer continuum.
   c. A family member or significant other who survives the loss of a loved one to cancer.
   d. An individual who has complete response to cancer therapy.

2. According to Mullan's "seasons of survival," the acute stage starts at the moment of diagnosis and:
   a. Ends when remission occurs.
   b. Ends before the initial treatment.
   c. Continues through the initial treatment.
   d. Continues through the completion of the initial treatment.

3. A cancer patient in the permanent stage of survival may be experiencing:
   a. Workplace discrimination.
   b. Fear of treatment side effects.
   c. The completion of cancer treatment.
   d. Isolation related to self-esteem issues.

4. Which chemotherapeutic agent is associated with inducing long-term side effects of cirrhosis and hepatic fibrosis?
   a. Bleomycin (Blenoxane).
   b. Chlorambucil (Leukeran).
   c. Dactinomycin (Cosmegen).
   d. Cisplatin (Platinol).

5. Factors contributing to the occurrence and frequency of late side effects of cancer therapy include all of the following EXCEPT:
   a. Extent of disease.
   b. Age of person at time of diagnosis.
   c. Coping strategies of the patient.
   d. Synergistic response of the treatment chosen.

6. A patient who has previously received radiation to his femur is at risk for which of the following long-term effects of the radiation?
   a. Tissue softening.
   b. Osteonecrosis.
   c. Bone demineralization.
   d. Kyphosis.

7. The psychological effects of cancer survival include the fear of reoccurrence as well as:
   a. Reluctance to transition from "being sick."
   b. Uneasiness regarding social situations.
   c. Anxiety related to follow-up health care.
   d. Increased depression related to the survival experience.

8. Which of the following prohibits workplace discrimination in federally funded agencies against cancer survivors?
   a. Public Information Act.
   b. Americans with Rehabilitation Act.
   c. The National Cancer Act of 1971.
   d. Federal Rehabilitation Act of 1973.

9. Insurance issues for an individual with a history of cancer include all of the following EXCEPT:
   a. Refusal of an application.
   b. Legal protection through COBRA Act of 1986.
   c. Increase in premiums.
   d. Reduction of benefits.

10. While waiting for a follow-up health appointment, a cancer survivor encounters another patient who is in the advanced stages of cancer and is not responding to treatment. The feeling the cancer survivor may experience is:
    a. Survivor phenomenon.
    b. Survivor sadness.
    c. Survivor guilt.
    d. Survivor acceptance.

11. Which of the following cancer survivor rights is not included in the Cancer Survivors' Bill of Rights?
    a. Pursuit of happiness.
    b. Equal job opportunities.
    c. Access to medical care.
    d. Assurance of individual coping.

12. An appropriate nursing intervention in supporting a cancer patient in the acute stage of survival is:
    a. Encouraging participation in a consumer policy group for health care.
    b. Encouraging annual health follow-ups.
    c. Assisting with obtaining information from the National Cancer Institute.
    d. Referring the patient to hospice services.

13. Existential and spiritual issues a cancer survivor may experience include all of the following EXCEPT:
    a. A renewed interest in financial issues.
    b. A richer sense of spirituality.
    c. A greater acceptance of self.
    d. A more intense desire for life.

*14. Survivorship and quality of life can be affected by a cancer patient developing cataracts. The development of cataracts can be caused by which of the following agents?
    a. Methotrexate (Rheumatrex).
    b. Ifosfamide (Ifex).
    c. Dexamethasone (Decadron).
    d. Etoposide (VePesid).

* Reflects advanced oncology nursing content

ANSWERS

1. **(b)**   The definition of cancer survivorship proposed by the National Coalition for Cancer Survivorship notes that survival begins at diagnosis of cancer and continues through to the final stages of life.

2. **(c)**   The acute stage of survival begins with diagnosis and extends through the initial treatment.

3. **(a)**   A patient in the permanent stage of survival will most likely be dealing with workplace discrimination including insurance issues.

4. **(c)**   Dactinomycin (Cosmegen) is the drug most associated with causing cirrhosis and hepatic fibrosis as a late effect of chemotherapy treatment.

5. **(d)**   Synergistic response of the treatment chosen does not affect late effects of cancer therapy.

6. **(b)**   Osteonecrosis and fractures are possible long-term effects from radiation therapy to the bone.

7. **(c)**   Psychological effects of survival include anxiety related to health care, a sense of vulnerability, and ambivalence about one's health status.

8. **(d)**   The Federal Rehabilitation Act of 1973 provides legal protection for cancer survivors who are discriminated against in a federally funded agency.

9. **(b)**   The COBRA (Consolidated Omnibus Budget Reconciliation) Act of 1986 only applies to employers who have at least 20 employees where medical coverage is mandated to be offered by the employer.

10. **(c)**   Survivor guilt is experienced when a cancer patient encounters other cancer patients who may not be doing as well.

11. **(d)**   Assurance of individual coping is not specifically outlined in the Cancer Survivors' Bill of Rights.

12. **(c)**   Assisting with the gathering of information is appropriate for the acute stage of survival.

13. **(a)**   Financial issues are related more to the psychosocial aspect of survival rather than the existential or spiritual.

*14. **(c)**   Steroids, such as dexamethasone (Decadron), can cause long-term or late effects of cataracts.

* Reflects advanced oncology nursing content

6

Sexuality

QUESTIONS

1. Which of the following is not an aspect of incorporating sexuality into patient care?
   a. Assessing sexual health.
   b. Educating patients.
   c. Sharing values regarding sexuality.
   d. Referring to appropriate resources.

2. Which theory related to human sexuality assists in planning nursing interventions?
   a. Johnson's behavioral model.
   b. Masters' and Johnson's sexuality theory.
   c. General systems theory.
   d. Human behavioral model.

3. Within the PLISSIT model, the "P" equates with:
   a. Provider.
   b. Permission.
   c. Program.
   d. Practice.

4. A patient receiving chemotherapy is using a diaphragm for birth control. It is important the nurse discuss which of the following with the patient?
   a. Transmission of sexually transmitted diseases.
   b. Body changes related to hormones.
   c. Contraception rate of the diaphragm.
   d. Infection control methods.

5. Since the first trimester is the greatest time of risk to a fetus, it is especially important to avoid which of the following antineoplastics?
   a. Mitotane (Lysodren).
   b. Vinblastine (Velban).
   c. Paclitaxel (Taxol).
   d. Methotrexate (Rheumatrex).

6. To reduce risk to a fetus, a cancer patient's diagnostic testing may be altered in all of the following ways EXCEPT:
   a. Shielding the fetus during diagnostic testing.
   b. Omitting diagnostic tests for late disease states.
   c. Substituting computed tomography for magnetic resonance imaging.
   d. Using ultrasonography instead of radiography.

7. During cancer therapy a pregnant patient has a higher risk for:
   a. Disseminated intravascular coagulation.
   b. Superior vena cava syndrome.
   c. Pleural effusion.
   d. Septic shock.

8. Which of the following is most related to fertility dysfunction in men?
   a. Combination chemotherapy regimen of ABVD (doxorubicin [Adriamycin], bleomycin, vinblastine, dacarbazine).
   b. Combination chemotherapy regimen of MOPP (mechlorethamine, vincristine [Oncovin], procarbazine, prednisone).
   c. Unilateral orchiectomy.
   d. Radiation therapy to the abdominal area.

9. Methods to preserve fertility with cancer treatment include all of the following EXCEPT:
   a. Reducing radiation treatment to 5 Gy.
   b. Oophoropexy.
   c. Sperm banking.
   d. Sperm retrieval from retrograde ejaculation.

10. A 38-year-old female is scheduled to receive pelvic radiation. Your patient teaching would include which of the statements?
   a. "Daily inspection of your vagina is important to prevent complications."
   b. "Vaginal intercourse is prohibited while you're being treated."
   c. "You will probably experience vaginal dryness."
   d. "You may notice increased elasticity of your vagina."

11. A 70-year-old male is being treated with 3 mg of oral diethylstilbestrol (DES) daily. The patient needs to be aware of which risk factor related to sexual function?
   a. Priapism.
   b. Gynecomastia.
   c. Increase in libido.
   d. Testicular edema.

12. A patient with early-stage testicular cancer is being treated with unilateral orchiectomy. The patient asks the nurse, "What is this surgery going to do to my sexual performance?" The best answer is:
   a. "Early ejaculation is highly associated with the type of surgery you had."
   b. "Don't worry, most impotence issues resolve over time."
   c. "Most likely you won't notice much change, since your surgery did not involve other organs or tissues."
   d. "You will probably notice erectile dysfunction, since your surgery involved genitourinary tissue."

13. A patient undergoing chemotherapy for lymphoma confides in the treatment nurse saying "My husband and I want sexual activity, but I fight being tired all the time. What can I do?" Which of the following should the nurse recommend?
   a. "You may want to drink a glass of wine to help you relax."
   b. "You and your husband may want to try a side-lying position for sexual activity."
   c. "A good meal will give you strength and stamina for sexual activity."
   d. "Napping after sexual activity will combat the feeling of fatigue."

14. A patient will be undergoing total abdominal hysterectomy tomorrow for cervical cancer. In assessing the patient's feelings about the potential impact of this procedure on her sexuality, the nurse should ask which of the following questions?
   a. "Most women have concerns about their sexuality after this surgery, do you have any concerns?"
   b. "All women experience sexual problems with this surgical procedure. Do you have any questions?"
   c. "Do you have any feelings regarding your sexuality related to this upcoming hysterectomy?"
   d. "Sexuality can be a problem with medical treatment. Do you have any problems?"

15. While engaging in sexual activity, a patient with a tracheostomy may experience production of secretions. What can the nurse suggest to the patient to deal with this?
   a. Wash the tracheostomy area with deodorizing antibacterial soap.
   b. Decrease fluid intake 4 hours before sexual activity.
   c. Place a thin piece of gauze over the tracheostomy.
   d. Use a scopolamine patch (Transderm Scōp).

16. Within the PLISSIT model, when is it appropriate for the oncology nurse to refer a patient to a sex therapist for intensive therapy?
    a. When the patient verbalizes anxiety and fear about body image and sex.
    b. When the patient wants to discuss alternative methods for sexual expression.
    c. When the patient inquires about masturbation techniques.
    d. When sexual dysfunction was a problem before the diagnosis of cancer occurred.

*17. Susan is a 28-year-old patient who has had a left mastectomy. At her first office visit, the nurse asks Susan how she is doing. Susan replies, "My appetite has not come back too well; I am not getting much sleep because I go to bed after my husband is asleep; and I am anxious to get back to work." Which of the following should the nurse pursue more in depth to support the patient's needs?
    a. Medication therapy for anorexia.
    b. Sexuality issues related to mastectomy.
    c. Insurance information related to her job.
    d. Medication therapy for insomnia.

* Reflects advanced oncology nursing content

ANSWERS

1. **(c)**   The sharing of sexual values is not appropriate when providing for holistic patient care.

2. **(a)**   Johnson's behavior model provides a basis for planning nursing interventions. It is based on seven integrated systems.

3. **(b)**   The "P" in the PLISSIT model stands for permission.

4. **(d)**   A patient receiving chemotherapy may become neutropenic. A higher risk of infection exists during neutropenia and the use of "invasive" devices, such as a diaphragm.

5. **(d)**   Antimetabolites such as methotrexate as well as alkylating agents are most often associated with malformations of a fetus.

6. **(c)**   Computed tomography causes exposure to radiation, which can cause adverse effects to a fetus.

7. **(a)**   While pregnant and undergoing cancer treatment, there is a higher risk of disseminated intravascular coagulation.

8. **(b)**   Combination chemotherapy with the MOPP regimen is associated with a fertility problem in 80% of male patients.

9. **(a)**   Radiation as minimal as 5 Gy can result in sterility.

10. **(c)**   Vaginal dryness is very common with pelvic radiation.

11. **(b)**   Gynecomastia is a distressing adverse effect of diethylstilbestrol (DES).

12. **(c)**   When simple, unilateral surgery is done to remove one testicle, usually no change in sexual function is noticed.

13. **(b)**   Side-lying, as a position for sexual activity, requires less effort and energy.

14. **(a)**   This question provides some basic information, while showing support for the patient who may experience sexual concerns.

15. **(c)**   Placing a thin piece of gauze over the tracheostomy will allow ventilation to occur but help to contain the secretions.

16. **(d)**   Long-standing or severe issues related to relationships and sexuality usually require the services of a therapist specifically trained in sex therapy.

*17. **(b)**   The data indicate the patient is avoiding intimacy with her husband. Exploring issues of sexuality is appropriate for a patient who has undergone a mastectomy.

---

* Reflects advanced oncology nursing content

CHAPTER 7

Symptom Management and Supportive Care: Dying and Death

QUESTIONS

1. Palliative care focuses on:
   a. Symptom management.
   b. Euthanasia care.
   c. Family involvement.
   d. Pain management.

2. In which of the following situations would hospice care not be indicated?
   a. A patient's cancer is progressing.
   b. A patient is receiving chemotherapy for metastatic cancer.
   c. A patient's cancer returns after a period of remission.
   d. A patient's prognosis is less than 6 months.

3. The central component of hospice care is:
   a. All hospice patients will experience dignified death at home.
   b. The patient's physician coordinates the care.
   c. A team approach directs hospice activity.
   d. The patient and or significant other are the focus of care.

4. A patient is experiencing severe pain from advanced cancer. Overall, the drug of choice to treat this patient's pain is:
   a. Oxycodone.
   b. Morphine sulfate.
   c. Hydromorphone (Dilaudid).
   d. Methadone (Dolophine).

5. A patient with prostate cancer metastatic to the bone is admitted to the hospital with severe pain unrelieved by pharmacologic methods. Which of the following is recommended for treatment:
   a. Iridium Ir 192.
   b. Heat and cold therapy.
   c. Radiostrontium 89.
   d. Transcutaneous electrical nerve stimulation.

6. A benefit of exercise for chronic pain is that it:
   a. Assists pain medications to work more effectively.
   b. Provides a relaxation response.
   c. Enhances mobilization of stiff joints.
   d. Provides body coordination.

7. A patient with metastatic breast cancer is experiencing extreme sedation as an effect from her pain management regimen. What can be added to the regimen to treat the sedation?
   a. A psychostimulant.
   b. A benzodiazepine.
   c. A steroid.
   d. An antidepressant.

8. When teaching a patient about implementing a pain control regimen, it is important for the nurse to instruct the patient about:
   a. Calling a pain clinic to treat severe pain.
   b. Using as-needed dosing to treat the pain.
   c. Contacting the physician if the pain is not totally relieved.
   d. Maintaining a written record of when pain medication and nondrug techniques were used.

9. An appropriate outcome for a patient in hospice is the:
    a. Patient incurs no adverse side effects of the pain management regimen.
    b. Physician is notified at the time of the patient's death.
    c. Patient experiences comfort at the time of death.
    d. Caregiver states strategies to treat pain.

10. A patient's hospice caregiver states, "He's not eating, so why is he still having bowel movements?" The nurse's best response is:
    a. "Eventually the bowels will shut down, but I don't know when that will be."
    b. "The intestines still produce some waste products even when a person is not eating."
    c. "The opioid medications will help to slow the process of bowel movements."
    d. "I know the bowel movements are distressing, but you must keep cleaning the patient to prevent skin breakdown."

11. Stool incontinence may occur as a result of metastatic disease causing spinal cord compression. What is the cause of the incontinence?
    a. Flaccid anal sphincter.
    b. Spastic anal sphincter.
    c. Irritable rectal sensation.
    d. Lower back pain.

12. To manage constipation in a patient starting on opioids, the nurse should initially suggest which of the following be used daily?
    a. Docusate (Colace) and bisacodyl (Dulcolax).
    b. Bisacodyl (Dulcolax) and lactulose (Chronulac).
    c. Docusate (Colace) and senna extract.
    d. Senna extract and sorbitol.

13. What is the role of oxygen therapy in a patient experiencing dyspnea?
    a. Provide comfort.
    b. Treat hypoxia.
    c. Prevent anxiety.
    d. Manage hypercapnia.

14. A patient with dyspnea will often report all of the following symptoms EXCEPT:
    a. A feeling of chest tightness.
    b. A sense of suffocation.
    c. A perception of distress.
    d. A sense of thoracic pain.

15. To minimize the discomfort of dyspnea, a patient can be advised to:
    a. Use pursed lip breathing.
    b. Maintain bedrest to conserve energy.
    c. Use nebulizer treatments.
    d. Engage in some exercise daily.

16. A caregiver tells the hospice nurse, "She won't eat, even though I prepare her favorite foods. What am I going to do?" Which of the following is the most appropriate nursing response by the nurse?
    a. "I will ask the physician to prescribe a medication to stimulate the patient's appetite."
    b. "The patient's disease has influenced her body's need and desire for food. Offer her food and fluids, but realize she often won't want them."
    c. "I suggest you offer liquid supplements. These provide high nutrition without you having to prepare them."
    d. "The patient may be trying to maintain control by not eating. Try to talk with your loved one to see if there are any underlying issues."

17. A patient with end-stage colon cancer is experiencing nausea with intermittent vomiting. Which of the following treatments would best serve this patient?
    a. Haloperidol (Haldol).
    b. Ondansetron (Zofran).
    c. Prochlorperazine (Compazine).
    d. Trimethobenzamide (Tigan).

18. Which of the following fluid and electrolyte disturbances does not precipitate nausea and vomiting in a patient with advanced cancer?
    a. Hypocalcemia.
    b. Syndrome of inappropriate antidiuretic hormone.
    c. Renal failure.
    d. Volume depletion.

19. A hospice patient is experiencing nausea and vomiting because of a bowel obstruction. Conservative management of the nausea and vomiting may be achieved with:
    a. Osmotic laxatives.
    b. Intravenous antiemetics.
    c. Nasogastric suction.
    d. A clear liquid diet.

20. Dehydration in terminally ill patients may cause all of the following positive outcomes EXCEPT:
    a. Decreased sensation resulting from dry mouth.
    b. Less vomiting.
    c. Decreased peripheral edema.
    d. Less incontinence.

21. A family member caring for a dying cancer patient should be informed that:
    a. The physician will make the decision regarding hydration therapy.
    b. Hydration is only used in extreme situations of dehydration.
    c. Dehydration is an expected event within the dying process.
    d. Dehydration may prolong the dying process.

22. The hospice on-call nurse receives a call from a family caregiver who stated her mother is suddenly seeing bugs on the wall, is confused as to her surroundings, and is irritable. The nurse suspects the patient is experiencing.
    a. Anxiety.
    b. Delirium.
    c. Agitation.
    d. Confusion.

23. In planning care for a cancer patient experiencing restlessness, it is important for the nurse to do all of the following EXCEPT:
    a. Continue medication doses as prescribed.
    b. Do not leave the patient unattended.
    c. Keep the room well-lit.
    d. Monitor for safety problems, such as a bed rail left down.

24. A patient's wife expresses concern about her dying husband's statements of "I have to go to the store now." In assisting the patient's wife to understand the dying process, the nurse should inform her that:
    a. Phrases related to leaving on a trip are common in dying persons.
    b. Restlessness can be treated with sedatives.
    c. The patient is trying to fight death.
    d. Decreased circulation to the brain often causes delirium.

25. A patient is dying with metastatic cancer after all treatment has been discontinued. The patient's breathing pattern is somewhat labored with moist sounds. The patient's daughter asks the nurse "Isn't there something you can do to help with her breathing?" The nurse's best intervention is:
    a. Suction the patient so that the patient's daughter knows all interventions were performed.
    b. Explain to the daughter that suctioning is not performed in dying patients.
    c. Reposition the patient, elevate the head of the bed, provide a cool compress.
    d. Assess the patient's vital signs and provide oral care.

26. A caregiver for an imminently dying home hospice patient needs to be instructed to do which of the following first?
    a. Call the hospice nurse when the patient dies.
    b. Call the hospice physician when the patient dies.
    c. Notify the funeral home.
    d. Call the county coroner.

27. A young leukemia patient has been actively dying for 24 hours. The nurse suggests which of the following to the patient's mother to support the death experience?
    a. Instruct her on how to provide medications to ease the patient's death.
    b. Inform the patient's mother that she may need to verbally tell the patient it's okay to let go and pass on.
    c. Encourage her to sit at the patient's bedside until death occurs.
    d. Tell her to make sure a chaplain is present at the time of death.

28. In assessing a patient for spiritual distress, an appropriate question would be:
    a. "What meaning do you give the situation you're in?"
    b. "What religious denomination do you follow?"
    c. "In your life, what have you done?"
    d. "Do you want to see a chaplain?"

29. The nurse formulates a nursing diagnosis of spiritual distress related to having a terminal illness. An appropriate goal for this patient would be to:
    a. Reflect on past accomplishments.
    b. Participate in practices that are spiritually supportive.
    c. Seek out a chaplain for spiritual guidance.
    d. Attend chapel services once a week.

30. Physical manifestations of grief related to the death of a loved one may include all of the following EXCEPT:
    a. Anxiety.
    b. Weight loss.
    c. Heart palpitations.
    d. Exhaustion.

*31. Mr. Cox has become increasingly dehydrated over the past 3 days. Which of the following signs is a positive effect of dehydration?
    a. Decreased abdominal girth.
    b. Increased gastric secretions.
    c. Increased renal perfusion.
    d. Improved skin turgor.

*32. For 5 months, Mary has been providing care in her home for her brother who has advanced lung cancer. Last month, Mary's husband of 25 years died of a sudden myocardial infarction. Knowing Mary is at risk for developing complicated grief, which of the following poses the least risk to Mary?
    a. Multiple losses.
    b. Social isolation.
    c. History of mental illness.
    d. Caregiver role strain.

*33. A patient's metastatic carcinoma of the lung has not responded to radiation therapy. The patient also has a history of chronic obstructive pulmonary disease. The hospice nurse is planning to visit the patient today for admission to hospice. Patient assessment will most likely reveal the patient is experiencing:
    a. Dyspnea.
    b. Ascites.
    c. Pleural friction rub.
    d. Peripheral edema.

*34. A 92-year-old patient with metastatic melanoma was found wandering the halls of the hospice unit calling out to his sons who were not present. As the nurse guided him back to his room, he became agitated, stating, "When are we going to Tallahassee?" The patient is receiving morphine (Roxanol) 20 mg PO every 4 hours for pain. He denies pain at this time. Which of the following agents is appropriate to add to the patient's medication regimen?
    a. Midazolam (Versed).
    b. Secobarbital (Seconal).
    c. Haloperidol (Haldol).
    d. Hydromorphone (Dilaudid).

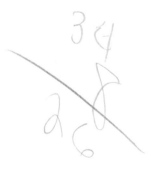

* Reflects advanced oncology nursing content

ANSWERS

1. **(a)** The overall goal of palliative care focuses on symptom management.

2. **(b)** Hospice care would not take place if a patient continued chemotherapy treatment for metastatic cancer.

3. **(d)** The most important central component of hospice care is focus of care on the patient as well as the family or other significant other.

4. **(b)** Morphine sulfate is the drug of choice to treat severe cancer pain.

5. **(c)** Radiostrontium 89 is a radiopharmaceutical used to treat pain not responsive to other treatments.

6. **(c)** Exercise assists with mobilizing stiff muscles and joints.

7. **(a)** A psychostimulant may offset the sedating effects of a pain management regimen.

8. **(d)** The patient or caregiver needs to maintain a record of pain management techniques, including medications or nondrug methods used.

9. **(c)** An appropriate outcome for a hospice patient is that the patient is comfortable at the time of death.

10. **(b)** It is important to provide factual information to answer a caregiver's question.

11. **(a)** A flaccid anal sphincter can be the result of spinal cord compression, which results in bowel incontinence.

12. **(d)** Senna extract and sorbitol.

13. **(a)** In dyspneic cancer patients, oxygen therapy provides comfort. It usually does not provide physiologic treatment of respiratory disorders.

14. **(d)** Usually thoracic pain is not a common subjective symptom reported with dyspnea.

15. **(a)** Pursed lip breathing may facilitate better gas exchange. This breathing technique can also relieve the sensation of dyspnea.

16. **(b)** A hospice patient usually has a disease process that has affected the body to the extent where anorexia is common. The body is not functioning in the same manner, thus food and fluids are not desired by the patient.

17. **(c)** Prochlorperazine (Compazine) is effective in terminal illness to treat nausea and vomiting.

18. **(a)** Hypocalcemia does not generally induce nausea and vomiting.

19. **(d)** Use of diet modification is a conservative approach to treat a hospice patient's nausea and vomiting related to bowel obstruction.

20. **(a)** Dry mouth remains a major problem with dehydration.

21. **(c)** Dehydration is an expected event with dying.

22. **(b)** Delirium is characterized by its acute onset and the symptoms of hallucinations, disorientation, and restlessness.

23. **(a)** The modification or discontinuation of medications may be needed to minimize restlessness.

24. **(a)** Mental changes are common with the dying. Comments that allude to trips, leaving, or deceased persons are common.

25. **(c)** These interventions support palliative care of the dying.

26. **(a)** The hospice nurse needs to be notified first at the time of a patient's death.

27. **(b)** Encouraging a significant other to give the dying person permission to die may support an easier death experience.

28. **(a)** This open-ended question will elicit information about what the person perceives as relevant to his or her spirituality.

29. **(b)** Spiritual practices that support a patient are an appropriate goal for the diagnosis of spiritual distress.

30. **(a)** Even though anxiety may be a component of grief, it is not a physical manifestation.

*31. **(a)** Positive effects of dehydration include decreased urine output, leading to less incontinence, decreased gastric secretions, less vomiting, less pulmonary secretions, decreased abdominal girth, and less peripheral edema.

*32. **(c)** It is not known if Mary has any history of mental illness, thus it is difficult to discern this to be a risk factor for her.

*33. **(a)** Causes of dyspnea in patients with advanced cancer include metastatic carcinoma of the lung, previous radiation therapy, and coexisting chronic obstructive pulmonary disease.

*34. **(c)** Haloperidol (Haldol) may help to relieve the patient's agitation.

---

* Reflects advanced oncology nursing content

Symptom Management and Supportive Care: Rehabilitation and Resources

QUESTIONS

1. The goal of rehabilitation for people with cancer is:
   a. Reintegration into the workplace.
   b. Achievement of optimal functioning.
   c. Restoration of function to previous levels.
   d. Coordination of resources to prevent complications of cancer.

2. Six months ago a young female underwent a right above-the-knee amputation to treat a stage II osteosarcoma. She is now adjusting to a leg prosthesis. What specific type of rehabilitation is this patient most likely receiving?
   a. Preventive rehabilitation.
   b. Restorative rehabilitation.
   c. Supportive rehabilitation.
   d. Palliative rehabilitation.

3. Which of the following is not a barrier to rehabilitation for cancer?
   a. Lack of available resources.
   b. Managed care health plans.
   c. Cancer viewed as a chronic illness.
   d. Limited community support.

4. A patient's coping strategies and self-concept are data recorded in which section of a rehabilitation assessment database?
   a. Psychosocial section.
   b. Demographic section.
   c. Physical section.
   d. Biographic section.

5. A nurse is working with a cancer patient to improve independence in activities of daily living. Which of the following is an appropriate nursing intervention?
   a. Always involve a family member with the rehabilitation sessions.
   b. Refer the patient to a community support group after rehabilitation is complete.
   c. Provide positive reinforcement for skills achieved.
   d. Inform the patient of rehabilitation plans made by the physician.

6. A cancer patient with financial concerns would best be served by a/an:
   a. Bank representative.
   b. Patient advocate.
   c. Oncology nurse.
   d. Social worker.

7. Which of the following is a rehabilitation resource person for a high school student returning to school after undergoing several weeks of cancer treatment?
   a. Occupational therapist.
   b. School counselor.
   c. Home health aid.
   d. Psychiatric nurse specialist.

8. An example of a local agency that may assist a cancer patient with nonmedical needs is the:
   a. Legal Aid Society.
   b. Community Hospital Network.
   c. American Association of Retired Persons.
   d. Citizens Advisory Team.

9. Which of the following is a primary nursing diagnosis for a patient with lung cancer who is participating in supportive rehabilitation?
    a. Body image disturbance.
    b. Activity intolerance.
    c. Powerlessness.
    d. Altered thought process.

10. An office oncology nurse is interested in obtaining information related to the experience of living with cancer. Which is the most appropriate periodical?
    a. *Seminars in Oncology Nursing.*
    b. *Ca—A Cancer Journal for Clinicians.*
    c. COPE.
    d. *Oncology Nursing Forum.*

11. A colon cancer patient is reluctant to attend support groups or educational classes about his disease, yet he has indicated the need for information and guidance. The most appropriate referral would be:
    a. Can Surmount.
    b. Make Today Count.
    c. National Coalition for Cancer Survivorship.
    d. I Can Cope.

12. A newly diagnosed cancer patient is searching for in-depth data regarding disease statistics and treatment plans. Where will the patient most likely find this information?
    a. American Cancer Society.
    b. Cancer Information Service.
    c. Cancer Care, Inc.
    d. National Cancer Information Network.

13. Which of the following resources would be most appropriate for a patient diagnosed with multiple myeloma?
    a. United Cancer Council.
    b. The Wellness Community.
    c. Leukemia Society of America.
    d. American Cancer Society.

*14. During an admission interview, the rehabilitation nurse notes tension among the patient's family members. The family members tell the nurse that the family has always had problems getting along. The nurse realizes that to meet the patient's rehabilitation goals, the nursing care plan needs to:
    a. Schedule all rehabilitation sessions when the family members are at work.
    b. Be aware of the family discord, and concentrate on the rehabilitation goals of the patient.
    c. Include a referral to a psychiatrist for a family evaluation.
    d. Plan care conferences for the family to resolve their issues.

*15. A 38-year-old woman with breast cancer is inquiring about counseling and education programs about breast cancer for herself and her best friend. The nurse suggests:
    a. The Oley Foundation.
    b. The Women's Cancer Network.
    c. Y-ME.
    d. The Breast Cancer Alliance.

* Reflects advanced oncology nursing content

ANSWERS

1. **(b)**   Rehabilitation for individuals with cancer is a process where optimal functioning and wellness is the goal.

2. **(b)**   Since the goal with amputation for early sarcoma is cure, this patient's rehabilitation is geared toward full functioning with total recovery expected.

3. **(c)**   Cancer is a chronic illness, but it is usually viewed as a terminal illness, which deters the concept of rehabilitation.

4. **(a)**   Psychosocial data for a rehabilitation assessment data base includes information such as personal characteristics, family functioning, and social needs.

5. **(c)**   Positive reinforcement builds confidence and facilitates achievement of rehabilitation goals.

6. **(d)**   A social worker can assist a cancer patient in discussing and dealing with financial concerns.

7. **(b)**   Rehabilitation resource people for reentry to school may include teachers, school counselors, social workers, and school nurses.

8. **(a)**   The Legal Aid Society may assist with nonmedical needs.

9. **(b)**   Activity intolerance is a primary nursing diagnosis for a patient with lung cancer who is participating in rehabilitation to prevent further complications.

10. **(c)**   COPE provides information about adapting to cancer on a daily basis.

11. **(a)**   Can Surmount is a program provided by the American Cancer Society in which volunteers visit patients with cancer to provide education and support.

12. **(b)**   The Cancer Information Service, sponsored by the National Cancer Institute, provides a wide range of data regarding cancer and treatments.

13. **(c)**   The Leukemia Society of America focuses on providing information and support to patients with hematologic diseases, such as multiple myeloma.

*14. **(b)**   Long-standing relationship patterns cannot be changed in a short period of time. Thus, it's important to be aware of the family tensions and concentrate on the rehabilitation goals of the patient.

*15. **(c)**   Y-ME is a national organization for breast cancer information and support that offers self-help support groups, counseling, and educational programs.

* Reflects advanced oncology nursing content

9

Symptom Management and Supportive Care: Therapies and Procedures

QUESTIONS

1. A short-term venous catheter inserted peripherally would be placed into the:
    a. External jugular vein.
    b. Cephalic vein.
    c. Internal jugular vein.
    d. Subclavian vein.

2. One purpose of the Dacron cuff in a tunneled long-term venous catheter is to:
    a. Serve as a barrier to infection.
    b. Minimize fibrin sheath formation.
    c. Anchor the catheter to the venous wall.
    d. Eliminate the need to use heparin for catheter irrigations.

3. What is a major complication with a peripherally inserted central catheter?
    a. Air embolism.
    b. Thrombosis.
    c. Malposition.
    d. Infection.

4. Which of the following is not an appropriate use for a long-term venous catheter?
    a. Frequent blood support therapy.
    b. Ongoing home total parenteral nutrition (TPN) therapy.
    c. Continuous chemotherapy infusions.
    d. Once-a-month blood sampling.

5. Urokinase was allowed to dwell 60 minutes in an occluded implanted access port. The nurse attempts to restore patency without success. The nurse's next action should be to:
    a. Instill 5,000 IU of urokinase.
    b. Instill 5,000 U of heparin.
    c. Instill 10,000 U of low molecular heparin.
    d. Instill 5 cc of normal saline.

6. Every morning when drawing blood from a patient's Hickman catheter, the nurse has to have the patient raise his arms and cough to be able to aspirate blood for the sampling. The nurse suspects the causative factor for the situation is:
    a. A fibrin sheath.
    b. The catheter is lodged against a vessel.
    c. The catheter is pinched between the clavicle and a rib.
    d. The catheter collapses secondary to excessive positive pressure.

7. Use of a 5-cc syringe to irrigate a Groshong catheter can result in catheter:
    a. Leakage.
    b. Constriction.
    c. Migration.
    d. Rupture.

8. A patient with hepatic cancer is to receive chemotherapy directly to the tumor area. Which vascular access device should be used?
    a. Peritoneal catheter.
    b. Arterial catheter.
    c. Abdominal catheter.
    d. Tunneled long-term venous catheter.

9. A nurse suspects a patient's venous access device is occluded by lipids. What agent should be used to restore patency?
   a. Normal saline.
   b. Hydrochloric acid.
   c. Ethyl alcohol.
   d. Sodium bicarbonate.

10. In teaching a patient how to prevent small holes and tracks from forming on a central venous access catheter, the nurse instructs the patient to do all of the following EXCEPT:
    a. Clamp the catheter properly.
    b. Avoid the use of sharp objects near the catheter.
    c. Move the clamp position on the catheter daily.
    d. Tape the catheter securely to the body.

11. The nurse knows a patient has understood discharge instructions about infection control of a long-term venous catheter when the patient states:
    a. "I will carefully perform my daily dressing exactly as you showed me."
    b. "It's important to wash my hands before and after irrigating the catheter."
    c. "I will check my temperature daily."
    d. "I will observe for drainage around the catheter site."

12. Upon entering a patient's room, the nurse finds the patient confused, short of breath, diaphoretic, and pale. The patient's pajamas are soaked with intravenous solution and the IV tubing is disconnected from the patient's tunneled central venous access device. The nurse's initial action is to:
    a. Elevate the head of the bed to 60°.
    b. Notify the physician.
    c. Place the patient on his left side in the bed.
    d. Clamp the IV tubing where the solution is infusing.

13. The third day into a 5-day regimen of continuous fluorouracil (5-FU) infusion via an implanted venous access port, the patient calls the office nurse and states she is experiencing intense pain at the port site and the area appears swollen. The nurse suspects which of the following has occurred?
    a. Pinch-off syndrome.
    b. Dislodgement of the port access needle.
    c. Erosion of the port septum.
    d. Infection at the port site.

14. A patient is receiving subcutaneous morphine for pain control. What type of infusion system is most appropriate?
    a. A large-volume controller device.
    b. A small-volume intermittent syringe device.
    c. A variable-flow controller pump.
    d. A small-volume programmable pump.

15. A cancer patient with intractable nausea and intermittent vomiting is receiving antiemetic therapy into an implanted port via continuous infusion from a portable pump. Over the last 2 hours, the patient has begun experiencing severe nausea with vomiting. The least likely cause of the patient's symptoms is:
    a. Migration of the implanted port.
    b. Leaking infusion tubing.
    c. Occlusion of the port needle.
    d. Mechanical failure of the pump.

16. Which of the following lab values indicates the need for the infusion of a blood product?
    a. Hemoglobin, 9 g/dL.
    b. Platelets, 32,000/mm^3.
    c. Hematocrit, 37%.
    d. Fibrinogen, 140 mg/dL.

17. On numerous occasions, a patient experienced febrile reactions to packed red blood cell transfusion. The nurse expects the patient will receive which type of blood component the next time the patient needs a transfusion for anemia?
    a. Denatured packed red blood cells.
    b. Leukocyte-poor packed red blood cells.
    c. Plasma-poor packed red blood cells.
    d. Frozen packed red blood cells.

18. A patient with leukemia is to receive HLA–matched platelets. Why is the patient receiving this type of platelet product?
    a. The patient's myelosuppression is severe.
    b. The patient experiences severe rigors with platelet infusions.
    c. The patient has experienced febrile reactions with previous platelet transfusions.
    d. The patient has demonstrated a refractory response to prior platelet infusion.

19. A patient is to receive two units of fresh frozen plasma. The nurse can expect to premedicate the patient with:
    a. Acetaminophen.
    b. Hydrocortisone.
    c. Meperidine.
    d. Acetylsalicylic acid.

20. Which of the following infusion rates is recommended for the administration of factor VIII to a patient with hemophilia A?
    a. Infuse over 2 hours.
    b. Infuse over 1 hour.
    c. Infuse over 30 minutes.
    d. Infuse rapidly.

21. A patient is receiving one unit of packed red blood cells. Thirty minutes into the infusion the patient begins to complain of chills, headache, and muscle aches. Which transfusion reaction is the patient most likely experiencing?
    a. Delayed hemolytic.
    b. Febrile, nonhemolytic.
    c. Allergic.
    d. Acute hemolytic.

22. When a nurse suspects a transfusion reaction, the initial nursing intervention is to:
    a. Notify the physician.
    b. Administer diphenhydramine.
    c. Keep the intravenous line open with normal saline.
    d. Stop the infusion.

23. Common electrolyte imbalances related to cancer-induced nutritional disturbances include all of the following EXCEPT:
    a. Hypophosphatemia.
    b. Hyperuricemia.
    c. Hyponatremia.
    d. Hypercalcaemia.

24. A nutritional outcome for a patient with advanced liver cancer would be:
    a. Maintain current weight.
    b. Gain one-half pound per week.
    c. Return to ideal body weight.
    d. Normalize albumin levels.

25. If a patient with cancer is experiencing an alteration in protein metabolism, which of the following processes does not occur?
    a. Protein synthesis decreases.
    b. Protein uptake by a tumor decreases.
    c. Protein degradation increases.
    d. Muscle protein breakdown decreases.

26. Anthropometric measurements may be used to assess a patient's nutritional status. Which of the following is an anthropometric measurement?
    a. Body surface area.
    b. Pre-albumin level.
    c. Mid-arm length.
    d. Albumin level.

27. A patient with colon cancer underwent a left hemicolectomy 3 weeks ago. The patient has had difficulty maintaining adequate oral intake to meet his metabolic needs for healing. Which of the following nutritional support methods is most appropriate for this patient?
    a. Nasogastric feeding tube.
    b. Jejunostomy.
    c. Total parenteral nutrition via central access.
    d. Total parenteral nutrition via peripheral access.

28. After receiving a bolus tube feeding, which position is most appropriate to place a patient in to prevent aspiration?
    a. Bedrest with head of the bed elevated 60° for 2 hours.
    b. Left lateral with head of the bed elevated 45° for 15 minutes.
    c. Sitting in a chair for 1 hour.
    d. Bedrest with head of the bed elevated 30° for 20 minutes.

29. A common complication of enteral nutrition is diarrhea. All of the following are causes of diarrhea EXCEPT:
    a. Contaminated solution.
    b. Lactose intolerance.
    c. Antibiotics.
    d. Abrupt discontinuation of feeding.

30. A patient is receiving total parenteral nutrition (TPN) through a subclavian triple-lumen catheter. The TPN bag is empty and another bag is not yet ready in the pharmacy. The most appropriate nursing action is to:
    a. Assess the patient carefully for signs of hyperglycemia.
    b. Turn off the TPN and flush the triple lumen subclavian catheter.
    c. Infuse 10% dextrose solution until a new TPN bag can be hung.
    d. Infuse 50% dextrose solution until a new TPN bag arrives.

31. A patient is to be discharged home with continuous total parenteral nutrition (TPN) via a tunneled long-term venous catheter. Which of the following statements reflects further patient teaching is needed regarding complications of TPN therapy?
   a.   "If I experience chest pain or coughing, I will call my doctor."
   b.   "I expect to gain weight, so I can weigh once a week to monitor my progress."
   c.   "Every day I will check my catheter site for redness."
   d.   "Even though I don't like to prick my finger, I will do my blood sugar checks twice a day."

*32. A bedbound 66-year-old patient with pancreatic cancer had a left subclavian long-term tunneled catheter placed 30 minutes ago. While awaiting radiographic confirmation of catheter placement, the patient becomes restless, short of breath, and complains of chest pain radiating to the midback area. Patient assessment reveals tachycardia and absent breath sounds in the left lung. The nurse suspects the patient is experiencing:
   a.   Pleural effusion.
   b.   Pulmonary embolus.
   c.   Pneumothorax.
   d.   Air embolus.

*33. A patient with chronic lymphocytic leukemia has received many units of packed red blood cells over the past 5 years. The patient is now experiencing arrhythmias, peripheral edema, dyspnea, and hypertension. The nurse is aware that these symptoms represent iron overload, which is treated with:
   a.   Desmopressin (Stimate).
   b.   Deferoxamine (Desferal).
   c.   Dexrazoxane (Zinecard).
   d.   Dezocine (Dalgan).

*34. A patient with esophageal cancer started 3 days ago with continuous feedings through a gastrostomy. The patient is 1 week into an 8-week course of radiation treatment to the esophagus. The patient's white blood cell count is 1500/mm^3, platelet count 36,000/mm^3, K+ 3.5 mEq/L, and Na+ 135 mEq/L. The patient has a documented allergy to sulfite. Currently, the patient is experiencing frequent nausea. Which antiemetic should be administered?
   a.   Haloperidol (Haldol).
   b.   Thiethylperazine maleate (Torecan).
   c.   Metoclopramide (Reglan).
   d.   Dronabinol (Marinol).

---

* Reflects advanced oncology nursing content

ANSWERS

1. **(b)** The cephalic vein is accessed peripherally via the antecubital fossa.

2. **(a)** The Dacron cuff serves as a barrier to infection and also stabilizes the catheter within the subcutaneous tissue.

3. **(c)** Malposition is a major complication of peripherally inserted central catheters.

4. **(d)** Infrequent use of a long-term venous access device warrants the choice of a different method of venous access.

5. **(a)** Instilling a second dose of urokinase is an acceptable intervention to restore patency to the venous access device.

6. **(b)** The ability to draw blood from the Hickman catheter after the patient coughs and raises his arms indicates the catheter is lodged against a vein wall.

7. **(d)** A Groshong catheter can rupture due to maximal pressure being exceeded. Recommended syringe size to use with a Groshong catheter is 10 cc to 20 cc to reduce pressure on the catheter.

8. **(b)** Since the liver is highly vascular, the most appropriate delivery system for the chemotherapy would be an arterial catheter.

9. **(c)** Seventy percent ethyl alcohol will dissolve an occlusion caused by lipids.

10. **(d)** Taping the catheter securely will prevent catheter trauma and dislodgement, but it will do little to prevent the occurrence of pin holes and tracks.

11. **(a)** Even though all the statements list methods to monitor and minimize infection, the most important intervention a patient can do to control infection is to perform meticulous catheter site care.

12. **(c)** The patient is exhibiting signs and symptoms of an air embolism. Placing the patient on the left side may trap the air in the right atrium of the heart.

13. **(b)** Dislodgement of the port access needle will allow an intravenous solution to infuse into the port area causing pain and swelling.

14. **(d)** A small-volume programmable pump is most appropriate for a patient receiving subcutaneous morphine.

15. **(a)** Even though migration of an implanted port can occur, it is rare when trauma to the area has not occurred.

16. **(d)** Normal fibrinogen levels are 200 to 400 mg/dL; thus an infusion with cryoprecipitate is warranted.

17. **(b)** Leukocyte-poor red blood cells limit febrile reactions to packed red blood cells.

18. **(d)** Patients who have received multiple transfusions may become alloimmunized to random donor or single donor platelets, with the result being a poor response to platelet therapy. HLA–matched platelets may improve the patient's response to platelet therapy.

19. **(a)** Acetaminophen is an antipyretic used to prevent or minimize transfusion reactions.

20. **(d)** Factor VIII can be infused rapidly into a patient with hemophilia A.

21. **(b)** The signs and symptoms indicate a febrile, nonhemolytic transfusion reaction.

22. **(d)** The first action when a transfusion reaction is suspected is to stop the infusion.

23. **(a)** Hypophosphatemia is not a common electrolyte imbalance related to cancer-induced nutritional disturbances.

24. **(a)** Preventing further weight loss is an acceptable nutritional goal for a patient with advanced cancer.

25. **(d)** As a result of increased protein degradation, muscle protein is broken down, which leads to loss of muscle mass.

26. **(a)** Anthropometric measurements include body surface area, midarm circumference, skinfold thickness, height, and weight.

27. **(d)** Total parenteral nutrition via central access is the most appropriate.

28. **(c)** The most appropriate position to prevent aspiration from a bolus tube feeding is sitting up for 30 to 60 minutes.

29. (d)   Abrupt discontinuation of enteral feedings does not generally cause diarrhea.

30. (c)   If an infusion of total parenteral nutrition (TPN) is suddenly interrupted, an infusion of 10% dextrose at the same infusion rate of the TPN is needed to prevent sudden and potentially severe hypoglycemia.

31. (b)   Even though weight gain is considered a positive outcome for TPN therapy, weight gain can be caused by fluid overload. It is important for a patient to monitor weight status daily.

*32. (c)   The patient is exhibiting signs of a pneumothorax even though he does have risk factors for a pulmonary embolus (pancreatic cancer and immobility). The patient most likely experienced a pneumothorax from the insertion of the subclavian venous catheter.

*33. (b)   Deferoxamine (Desferal) chelates and removes accumulated iron via the kidneys.

*34. (c)   The nausea may be caused by delayed gastric emptying resulting from the newly initiated continuous gastrostomy feedings. Metoclopramide (Reglan) facilitates gastric emptying. Since the patient is neutropenic, Italoperidol (Italdol) should not be used since it can cause further hematologic compromise. Dronabinol (Marinol) is usually used for chemotherapy-related nausea. Patients with sulfite allergies should avoid thiethylperazine (Torecan).

* Reflects advanced oncology nursing content

CHAPTER 10

Symptom Management and Supportive Care: Pharmacologic Interventions

QUESTIONS

1. A patient's temperature is 100.7° F and the physician has ordered a fever workup. The nurse knows that all the following will be included in the workup EXCEPT:
   a. Blood culture.
   b. Urine culture.
   c. Saliva culture.
   d. Stool culture.

2. If a cancer patient has a history of herpes zoster, which of the following drugs should be added to an antibiotic regimen?
   a. Chloramphenicol (Chloromycetin).
   b. Acyclovir (Zovirax).
   c. Foscarnet (Foscavir).
   d. Itraconazole (Sporanox).

3. A neutropenic patient has not responded to 7 days of antibiotic treatment. The nurse suspects an infection caused by which of the following organisms?
   a. *Aspergillus* species.
   b. *Cryptococcus* species.
   c. *Histoplasma* species.
   d. *Torulopsis* species.

4. Which of the following is not a hematologic complication of antimicrobial therapy?
   a. Anemia.
   b. Neutropenia.
   c. Bleeding.
   d. Clotting.

5. The nurse is monitoring a patient receiving ampicillin (Omnipen). Which common side effect can the nurse expect?
   a. Hypertension.
   b. Headache.
   c. Hypokalemia.
   d. Hypercalcemia.

6. High-dose therapy with cefazolin (Ancef) can cause:
   a. Seizures.
   b. Skin rash.
   c. Diarrhea.
   d. Cross sensitivity.

7. Third-generation cephalosporins usually provide broader coverage of certain bacteria; however, a disadvantage of these antimicrobials is they can cause:
   a. Thrombocytosis.
   b. Leukopenia.
   c. Hyponatremia.
   d. Hyperuricemia.

8. An example of a drug in the β-lactam class of antimicrobials is:
   a. Norfloxacin (Noroxin).
   b. Levofloxacin (Levaquin).
   c. Imipenem/cilastatin (Primaxin).
   d. Imipramine (Tofranil).

9. Ciprofloxacin (Cipro), 500 mg po bid, has been ordered for a patient at home for the next 10 days. It is important to teach the patient to:
   a. Assess the oral mucosa every day since gingival bleeding and infection is common.
   b. Call the physician if nausea occurs, since this is an uncommon side effect.
   c. Take a double dose of the ciprofloxacin if a dose is missed during the 10 days.
   d. Avoid antacids 2 hours before and 2 hours after taking the ciprofloxacin.

10. When taking ofloxacin (Floxin), the nurse must teach the patient that:
    a. Blood sugar changes may occur.
    b. Liver function test results may be elevated.
    c. Transient leukopenia may occur.
    d. Hypocalcemia may occur.

11. A patient is being treated with amikacin sulfate. To which class of antibacterial agents does amikacin belong?
    a. Aminoglycosides.
    b. Extended spectrum penicillins.
    c. Cephalosporins.
    d. Monobactams.

12. Hearing loss, balance disturbances, and skin tingling are toxicities caused by which drug?
    a. Aztreonam (Azactam).
    b. Ticarcillin (Ticar).
    c. Tobramycin sulfate (Nebcin).
    d. Gentamicin sulfate (Garamycin).

13. Adrenal insufficiency can occur with which antifungal?
    a. Miconazole nitrate (Monistat-Derm).
    b. Ketoconazole (Nizoral).
    c. Clotrimazole (Lotrimin).
    d. Flucytosine (Ancobon).

14. An important parameter to assess and monitor in the patient receiving amphotericin B intravenously is:
    a. Increased serum creatinine level.
    b. Increased sodium level.
    c. Decreased white blood cell count.
    d. Decreased BUN level.

15. Reactions to ganciclovir (Cytovene) primarily affect which body systems?
    a. Hematologic and renal.
    b. Gastrointestinal (GI) and central nervous system.
    c. Hematologic and hepatic.
    d. Renal and hepatic.

16. Which factor must be considered when determining foscarnet (Foscavir) dosage for a 22-year-old with AIDS-related cytomegalovirus retinitis?
    a. Renal function.
    b. Age.
    c. Body weight.
    d. Liver function.

17. What is the most toxic reaction to chloramphenicol (Chloromycetin)?
    a. Seizures.
    b. Bone marrow suppression.
    c. Cardiomyopathy.
    d. Renal failure.

18. An antibacterial agent used to treat gram-positive bacteria is:
    a. Tetracycline (Achromycin).
    b. Vancomycin (Vancocin).
    c. Kanamycin (Kantrex).
    d. Metronidazole (Flagyl).

19. A patient is admitted with an *Escherichia coli* urinary tract infection. Which of the following drugs would be used to treat the urinary tract infection?
    a. Trimethoprim-sulfamethoxazole (Bactrim).
    b. Trimetrexate (Neutrexin).
    c. Erythromycin (E-Mycin).
    d. Clindamycin (Cleocin).

20. A body's primary defense against bacteria is often altered by:
    a. Noninvasive procedures.
    b. Fluid and electrolyte imbalances.
    c. Disruption of the skin.
    d. Steroid use.

21. The inflammatory process involves the production of:
    a. Lycopene.
    b. Lymph.
    c. Endotoxins.
    d. Prostaglandins.

22. Before starting a patient on aspirin therapy, the nurse assesses the patient's medical history. Which condition alerts the nurse to a contraindication for the aspirin therapy?
    a. Cardiac disease.
    b. Bleeding disorder.
    c. Renal malfunction.
    d. Pulmonary dysfunction.

23. Ketoprofen (Orudis) is what type of nonsteroidal anti-inflammatory?
    a. Propionic acid.
    b. Salicylate.
    c. Oxicam.
    d. Acetic acid.

24. A patient with advanced prostate cancer has bone metastases. Which of the following drugs would be used to treat the discomfort related to bone metastases?
    a. Acetaminophen (Tylenol).
    b. Morphine.
    c. Amitryptiline (Elavil).
    d. Indomethacin (Indocin).

25. An alternative drug for aspirin that can be prescribed for a patient with aspirin sensitivity is:
    a. Fenoprofen (Nalfon).
    b. Diclofenac (Voltaren).
    c. Choline magnesium trisalicylate (Trilisate).
    d. Sulindac (Clinoril).

26. The nurse should withhold a scheduled ketoralac tromethamine (Toradol) dose and notify the physician when which adverse reaction occurs?
    a. Diarrhea.
    b. Urinary frequency.
    c. Malaise.
    d. Severe GI pain.

27. An example of a long-acting corticosteroid is:
    a. Dexamethasone (Decadron).
    b. Hydrocortisone (Solu-Cortef).
    c. Methylprednisolone (Medrol).
    d. Prednisone (Sterapred).

28. An appropriate nursing intervention to reduce the complications of etodolac (Lodine) therapy is to instruct the patient to avoid:
    a. Stress.
    b. Eating raw vegetables.
    c. Sunlight.
    d. Crowds.

29. Which of the following agents has a higher frequency of anaphylactoid reactions?
    a. Ibuprofen (Motrin).
    b. Diclofenac (Voltaren).
    c. Salsalate (Disalcid).
    d. Tolmetin (Tolectin).

30. Which of the following is not a risk factor for renal failure related to NSAIDS?
    a. Advanced age.
    b. Existing renal dysfunction.
    c. Congestive heart failure.
    d. Pancreatitis.

31. Which adverse cardiovascular reaction can occur with nonsteroidal anti-inflammatory agents?
    a. Edema.
    b. Hypotension.
    c. Dysrhythmias.
    d. Palpitations.

32. During corticosteroid therapy, the nurse should monitor a patient for which adverse reaction?
    a. Fluid and electrolyte imbalances.
    b. Nausea and vomiting.
    c. Blurred vision.
    d. Skin rash.

33. An important outcome for a patient taking prednisone (Delta-Cortef) is that the patient:
- a. Remains free from infection.
- b. Avoids Cushing's syndrome.
- c. Recovers from an infectious process.
- d. Avoids hypoglycemia.

34. Nonsteroidal anti-inflammatory drugs can increase the effects of which of the following drugs?
- a. Diltiazem (Cardizem).
- b. Propranolol (Inderal).
- c. Phenytoin (Dilantin).
- d. Furosemide (Lasix).

35. Anticipatory nausea and vomiting is usually aggravated by:
- a. Stimulation of chemoreceptor trigger zone.
- b. Anxiety.
- c. Stimulation of the vestibular-cerebellar zone.
- d. Loneliness.

36. Which of the following chemotherapeutic agents has the highest emetogenic potential?
- a. Docetaxel (Taxotere).
- b. Bleomycin (Blenoanxe).
- c. Ifosfamide (Ifex).
- d. Dacarbazine (DTIC).

37. A health problem that may preclude the use of certain antiemetics is:
- a. Glaucoma.
- b. Hypertension.
- c. Diabetes.
- d. Pancreatitis.

38. A patient receiving etoposide (VP-16) and cisplatin (Platinol) therapy for lung cancer requests information about the best way to avoid nausea and vomiting. The nurse's best response would be:
- a. "Take the antiemetics only if you feel nauseated so that you don't become too sedated."
- b. "When your nausea subsides in the next day or so, you can take your antiemetics as needed."
- c. "It's important to maintain your antiemetics regimen around the clock for the next 4 days."
- d. "Take your antiemetics around the clock for the next 24 hours, then take the antiemetics every 6 hours as needed."

39. A common side effect of serotonin antagonists is:
- a. Tachycardia.
- b. Sedation.
- c. Headache.
- d. Dry mouth.

40. A patient is receiving metoclopramide (Reglan) as an antiemetic for chemotherapy. The patient begins to move his mouth awkwardly to the side. The best nursing intervention is to:
- a. Administer dexamethasone (Decadron).
- b. Administer diphenhydramine (Benadryl).
- c. Administer epinephrine.
- d. Administer lorazepam (Ativan).

41. Which of the following drugs belongs to the phenothiazine class of antiemetics?
    a. Prochlorperazine (Compazine).
    b. Droperidol (Inapsine).
    c. Granisetron (Kytril).
    d. Hydroxyzine (Vistaril).

42. When a patient is receiving chlorpromazine (Thorazine) as an antiemetic, the nurse should teach the patient how to minimize the effects of:
    a. Bradycardia.
    b. Dyspepsia.
    c. Diarrhea.
    d. Orthostatic hypotension.

43. Corticosteroids may cause which of the following side effects?
    a. Hiccoughs.
    b. Hypoglycemia.
    c. Hyperkalemia.
    d. Hypotension.

44. When dronabinol (Marinol) is used as an antiemetic, which of the following patients is most likely to experience enhanced adverse central nervous system reactions?
    a. A 25-year-old with lymphoma.
    b. A 13-year-old with sarcoma.
    c. A 66-year-old with colon cancer.
    d. A 40-year-old with breast cancer.

45. Which of the following patient statements indicates a need for further education regarding the use of hydroxyzine (Vistaril) as an antiemetic?
    a. "I need to drink small amounts of clear fluids frequently to help keep my mouth moist."
    b. "If I seem to have difficulty staying awake during the day, I will let my nurse know."
    c. "I cannot operate my woodworking machinery while using the medication."
    d. "I will still be able to enjoy my one glass of wine at night to help me sleep."

46. A patient with stomach cancer is admitted to the hospital after experiencing 3 days of vomiting. Physical assessment reveals muscle twitching and irregular pulse. The patient states "my fingers feel like pins and needles." Lab work reveals K + 2.9 mEq/L and blood gases show a pH of 7.46 and bicarbonate of 29 mEq/L. The nurse suspects the patient is experiencing:
    a. Metabolic acidosis.
    b. Metabolic alkalosis.
    c. Respiratory acidosis.
    d. Respiratory alkalosis.

47. A patient with metastic brain cancer takes phenobarbital (Barbita) to control seizures. Which of the following drugs should be avoided?
    a. Promethazine (Phenergan).
    b. Diphenhydramine (Benadryl).
    c. Thiethylperazine maleate (Torecan).
    d. Scopolamine (Transderm-Scōp).

48. Which of the following is an agonist-antagonist analgesic compound?
    a. Sufentanil citrate (Sufenta).
    b. Levorphanol tartrate (Levo-Dromoran).
    c. Buprenorphine hydrochloride (Buprenex).
    d. Tramadol (Ultram).

49. Which analgesic's effects are most likely to have a duration of 4 to 6 hours?
    a. Meperidine (Demerol).
    b. Morphine.
    c. Pentazocine (Talwin).
    d. Butorphanol (Stadol).

50. Opioid analgesics can cause which side effect?
    a. Hiccoughs.
    b. Urinary frequency.
    c. Photophobia.
    d. Miosis.

51. Which of the following is recommended for assessment of opioid-induced respiratory depression?
    a. Monitoring for apnea.
    b. Monitoring sedation level.
    c. Assessment of pulse oximetry.
    d. Assessment of blood gas results.

52. In checking a patient's medication record, the nurse notes that the patient is concomitantly using hydromorphone hydrochloride (Dilaudid) and cimetidine (Tagamet). The nurse can expect what type of an effect?
    a. Increased effect of the Dilaudid.
    b. Decreased effect of the Dilaudid.
    c. Increased effect of the Tagamet.
    d. Decreased effect of the Tagamet.

53. On a routine follow-up visit, a patient states, "The doctor says my blood pressure is pretty high. I had my blood pressure checked last week at the senior center, and it was also high. I don't understand it. I am taking captopril (Capoten). I am also taking my diclofenac (Voltaren) as prescribed." The nurse's best response is:
    a. "You are probably experiencing anxiety at the time your blood pressure is being taken. We'll need to devise a way for you to check your blood pressure at home."
    b. "Your pain medication may be affecting your blood pressure medication so that your blood pressure is elevated."
    c. "Are you sure you're taking your blood pressure medication correctly?"
    d. "You may be having some kidney problems, which will affect your blood pressure medication as well as your pain medication."

54. Symptoms of opioid withdrawal include all of the following EXCEPT:
    a. Diaphoresis.
    b. Hallucinations.
    c. Hypotension.
    d. Nausea.

55. Decreased absorption of analgesics may be caused by all of the following EXCEPT:
    a. Tube feedings.
    b. Cisapride (Propulsid).
    c. Gastrectomy.
    d. Loperamide (Imodium).

56. A nurse informs a patient that his opioid analgesics can cause hypotension. The nurse is aware that the side effects of hypotension are caused by:
    a.   Diuresis.
    b.   Arteriolar vasodilation.
    c.   Decreased stroke volume.
    d.   Decreased vessel elasticity.

57. Because Mr. Jones will be taking morphine elixir for cancer pain, he needs to be aware that it is important to notify the physician for which of the following side effects?
    a.   Diarrhea.
    b.   Increased coughing reflex.
    c.   Muscle twitching.
    d.   Urinary stress incontinence.

58. A teaching plan for a patient with advanced cancer using opioid therapy should include all of the following EXCEPT:
    a.   How to treat respiratory depression.
    b.   The management of constipation.
    c.   An explanation of tolerance and addiction.
    d.   How to measure and report pain.

59. Potential complications of psychotropic drugs include all of the following EXCEPT:
    a.   Hyperventilation.
    b.   Drug dependence.
    c.   Combative behavior.
    d.   Noncompliance.

60. In planning care for a Chinese patient experiencing anxiety, the nurse is aware of which of the following?
    a.   Initial therapy should include a neuroleptic medication with a higher starting dose than usually prescribed.
    b.   Amobarbital (Amytal) is a drug to provide adjunct therapy for this patient.
    c.   Therapy should begin with a lower dose than usually prescribed of a chosen benzodiazepine agent.
    d.   Secobarbital (Seconal) has a low tolerance profile, which makes this drug an appropriate choice for this patient.

61. A patient using secobarbital (Seconal) for severe insomnia reports feeling cold, weak, and nauseated. Further assessment reveals clammy, moist skin and a blood pressure of 80/50 mm Hg. The nurse suspects the patient is experiencing:
    a.   Extrapyramidal effects.
    b.   Barbiturate withdrawal.
    c.   Stevens-Johnson syndrome.
    d.   Barbiturate toxicity.

62. A patient with kidney cancer notifies the homecare nurse and states, "Since I started using that sleeping pill a few days ago, I just don't feel right. I can't stay awake in the daytime and I feel very on edge." The nurse expects the patient to report that he is taking:
    a.   Flurazepam.
    b.   Temazepam (Restoril).
    c.   Triazolam (Halcion).
    d.   Oxazepam (Serax).

63. A patient using triazolam (Halcion) is more likely to experience dose-related side effects if the patient has which disease?
   a. Renal disease.
   b. Liver disease.
   c. Lung disease.
   d. Heart disease.

64. A patient taking short-acting benzodiazepines to treat anxiety should receive instruction about which of the following self-care measures?
   a. Rise slowly when getting out of bed or chairs.
   b. Increase fiber foods in the diet.
   c. Void every 2 hours.
   d. Elevate feet when sitting.

65. A cancer patient with a history of alcohol abuse is admitted to the hospital for dehydration and vomiting. Which of the following medications will the physician order to minimize anxiety and alcohol withdrawal symptoms?
   a. Alprazolam (Xanax).
   b. Lorazepam (Ativan).
   c. Diazepam (Valium).
   d. Chlordiazepoxide hydrochloride (Librium).

66. A common side effect of the phenothiazine class of anti-anxiety drugs is:
   a. Hypertension.
   b. Extrapyramidal effects.
   c. Decreased libido.
   d. Hypothermia.

67. Teaching for a patient beginning fluphenazine (Prolixin) therapy should include:
   a. Information to restrict fluid intake to 1200 mL/day.
   b. Signs and symptoms of hypoglycemia.
   c. Information that the patient's urine may turn pink or maroon.
   d. Signs and symptoms of high blood pressure.

68. Mrs. Stevens has epilepsy and breast cancer. She is experiencing symptoms of anxiety. Which of the following drugs should NOT be prescribed for Mrs. Stevens?
   a. Haloperidol (Haldol).
   b. Clorazepate (Tranxene).
   c. Lorazepam (Ativan).
   d. Oxazepam (Serax).

69. Which of the following patients has a risk factor for the development of depression?
   a. A 68-year-old with stage I breast cancer.
   b. A 76-year-old with adequate pain management.
   c. A 34-year-old with remission from leukemia.
   d. A 39-year-old with Dukes' C colon cancer.

70. Mr. Stone began amitriptyline (Elavil) therapy 1 week ago for treatment of depression. He reports to you by phone that he is feeling somewhat better but he is distressed by his constant mouth dryness. The nurse's best response is:
   a. "Increasing your fluid intake will help with the mouth dryness, but you may want to discontinue the medication if the dryness is too bothersome."
   b. "Mouth dryness may diminish some as you continue with the medication, but try to suck sugarless candy and sip fluids during the day."
   c. "It sounds as if you're experiencing an adverse reaction. I'll speak to the physician about prescribing another medication for you."
   d. "I'm sure the mouth dryness is something you can accept now that you're feeling better from the medication."

71. Which of the following agents does not belong to the specific serotonin-reuptake inhibitors class of antidepressants?
   a. Trazodone (Desyrel).
   b. Fluoxetine (Prozac).
   c. Sertraline (Zoloft).
   d. Venlafaxine (Effexor).

72. A physician would need to switch a patient from valproate or valproic acid (Depakote) to a different anticonvulsant if which of the following conditions developed?
   a. Renal failure.
   b. Hepatic failure.
   c. Cardiac dysfunction.
   d. Pulmonary dysfunction.

73. A patient with metatastic lung cancer is admitted to the hospital with complaints of malaise and weakness. He last received radiation treatment 6 weeks ago. Lab work reveals a WBC count of $1000/mm^3$, hemoglobin level of 10 g/dL, and a platelet count of $20,000/mm^3$. What drug in his therapeutic regimen to control seizures and pain may be the cause of the patient's clinical situation?
   a. Oxycodone with aspirin (Percodan).
   b. Gabapentin (Neurotin).
   c. Fentanyl (Duragesic).
   d. Carbamazepine (Tegretol).

74. Both sargramostim (Leukine) and filgrastim (Neupogen) can cause which side effect?
   a. Nausea.
   b. Fever.
   c. Bone pain.
   d. Headache.

75. When treatment with erythropoietin (Procrit) is considered, which of the following conditions may contraindicate the proposed therapy?
   a. Uncontrolled hypertension.
   b. Renal failure.
   c. Bleeding disorder.
   d. Chronic obstructive pulmonary disease.

76. Which of the following chronic illnesses may be exacerbated by the use of growth factors?
   a. Osteoarthritis.
   b. Diabetes.
   c. Hypothyroidism.
   d. Asthma.

*77. Mrs. Stone is a 65-year-old Hispanic woman with a granulocyte count of 800/mm^3. She has a history of congestive heart failure, chronic obstructive pulmonary disease, and diabetes mellitus. Her medication history includes digoxin (Lanoxin), potassium (K-Lyte), prednisone, and acarbose (Precose). Which of the above data shows that this patient is at risk for altered phagocytic defenses in relation to the development of infection?
   a. Prednisone and granulocytopenia.
   b. Diabetes mellitus and digoxin (Lanoxin).
   c. Acarbose (Precose) and chronic obstructive pulmonary disease.
   d. Female gender and congestive heart failure.

*78. Mr. Barnes is allergic to penicillin. He has a positive culture for *Klebsiella* species. The nurse is aware that 5% to 15% of patients allergic to penicillin G have a cross sensitivity to:
   a. Ciprofloxacin (Cipro).
   b. Tobramycin (Nebcin).
   c. Cephalothin (Keflin).
   d. Imipenem/cilastin (Primaxin).

*79. Mr. Banks has ototoxicity from previous high-dose cisplatin (Platinol) therapy. He also has a history of dizziness caused by middle ear infections, vertigo, and lower extremity phlebitis. He has a culture positive for *Streptococcus fecalis*. According to Mr. Banks' history, which of the following antimicrobial agents would be contraindicated?
   a. Vancomycin (Vanocin).
   b. Ampicillin (Omnipen).
   c. Methicillin sodium (Staphcillin).
   d. Carbenicillin indanyl sodium (Geocillin).

*80. A patient has a primary brain tumor that requires a long-acting corticosteroid for its anti-inflammatory properties. Which of the following is a long-acting corticosteroid?
   a. Hydrocortisone.
   b. Methylprednisolone (Medrol).
   c. Prednisone.
   d. Dexamethasone (Decadron).

*81. A patient with stage IV prostate cancer with bone metastases is under hospice care. The patient has severe episodes of congestive heart failure, which decrease his quality of life. Which of the following would be contraindicated in treating bone metastases because of its side effect of fluid retention?
   a. Indomethacin (Indocin).
   b. Naproxen (Naprosyn).
   c. Ibuprofen (Motrin).
   d. Piroxicam (Feldene).

*82. Ms. Weeks has hard-to-control psychomotor epilepsy. She is prescribed phenytoin (Dilantin) to control her disease process. Which of the following phenytoin (Dilantin) preparations should not be used due to its erratic absorption?
   a. Suspension.
   b. Intravenous solution.
   c. Capsules.
   d. Suppositories.

---

* Reflects advanced oncology nursing content

*83. A patient with anxiety has been treated with alprazolam (Xanax). Before the initiation of drug therapy, the patient's blood pressure was 136/72 mm Hg. After a second dose of alprazolam (Xanax), her blood pressure is 106/68 mm Hg. The nurse's next action should be to:
a. Continue to give the medication.
b. Monitor for extrapyramidal effects.
c. Hold the medication.
d. Increase the patient's oral fluids to 200 mL/hr.

*84. Mr. Hazelwood has been prescribed dronabinol (Marinol) for anti-emetic therapy. Which of the following vital sign findings would be indicative of an adverse reaction to this medication?
a. Orthostatic hypotension.
b. Fever.
c. Bradycardia.
d. Hypertension.

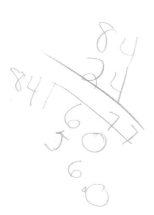

ANSWERS

1. **(c)** Saliva is not helpful in a fever workup; however, sputum would be collected.

2. **(b)** Acyclovir (Zovirax) is an antiviral that is used to treat herpes zoster.

3. **(a)** The most common organisms that cause fungal infections in neutropenic patients are *Aspergillus* and *Candida* species.

4. **(d)** Clotting is usually not a hematologic complication incurred with antimicrobial therapy.

5. **(c)** Hypokalemia is a common side effect of taking ampicillin and other penicillins.

6. **(a)** High doses of cefazolin can cause seizures and renal failure.

7. **(b)** Transient leukopenia can be caused by third-generation cephalosporins.

8. **(c)** Imipenem/cilastatin (Primaxin) belongs to the β-lactam class of antimicrobials.

9. **(d)** Antacids decrease the absorption of ciprofloxacin (Cipro). The antacids should not be given within 2 hours of taking ciprofloxacin.

10. **(a)** Ofloxacin (Floxin) is associated with changes in blood sugar.

11. **(a)** Amikacin is an aminoglycoside.

12. **(d)** Gentamicin sulfate can cause vestibular toxicity, including hearing loss and balance problems. Also, skin tingling may occur.

13. **(b)** Adrenal insufficiency has been reported with ketoconazole use.

14. **(a)** Renal failure is common with amphotericin B infusions, so monitoring for an increased serum creatinine level is important to detect renal failure promptly.

15. **(c)** Common reactions to ganciclovir (Cytovene) are neutropenia, thrombocytopenia, and increases in liver function tests.

16. **(a)** Renal function is important when considering dosages for foscarnet (Foscavir).

17. **(b)** Chloramphenicol (Chloromycetin) causes bone marrow suppression.

18. **(b)** Vancomycin is used to treat gram-positive bacterial infections.

19. **(a)** Trimethoprim-sulfamethoxazole is active against *E. coli*.

20. **(c)** Skin serves as the first line of defense against bacteria. Disruption of the skin can be caused by surgery, invasive procedures, extravasation, burns, and stomatitis.

21. **(d)** Prostaglandins are produced with inflammation and are associated with causing pain.

22. **(b)** Aspirin is contraindicated in patients with bleeding disorders, because aspirin affects platelet aggregation and prolongs bleeding time.

23. **(a)** Ketoprofen (Orudis) belongs to the propionic acid class of nonsteroidal anti-inflammatory agents.

24. **(d)** Indomethacin (Indocin) is useful in treating pain related to bone metastases.

25. **(c)** Choline magnesium trisalicylate (Trilisate) has no antiplatelet effect and can be given to patients with a sensitivity to aspirin.

26. **(d)** Severe GI pain may indicate bleeding. GI bleeding is a severe adverse reaction of ketorolac tromethamine (Toradol).

27. **(a)** Dexamethasone (Decadron) is a long-acting corticosteroid.

28. **(c)** Etodolac (Lodine) can cause photosensitivity reactions, thus avoiding the sun is important.

29. **(d)** Tolmetin (Tolectin) is associated with a higher frequency of anaphylactoid reactions.

30. **(d)** Pancreatitis is not a risk factor associated with renal failure caused by nonsteroidal anti-inflammatories.

31. **(a)** Fluid retention leading to edema and hypertension can occur.

32. **(a)** Fluid and electrolyte imbalances are common with corticosteroid therapy. Monitoring of fluid and electrolytes may minimize severe complications.

33. **(a)** Remaining free of infection is an important outcome for a patient taking prednisone, since immunosuppression is a common effect of the therapy.

34. **(c)** Nonsteroidal anti-inflammatory agents increase the effects of phenytoin (Dilantin).

35. **(b)** Anticipatory nausea and vomiting is a conditioned response and it is aggravated by anxiety.

36. **(d)** Dacarbazine (DTIC) has a more than 90% chance of causing nausea and vomiting in patients receiving it.

37. **(a)** Glaucoma is a condition that prevents the use of numerous antiemetics, such as prochlorperazine (Compazine) and promethazine (Phenergan).

38. **(c)** Since cisplatin (Platinol) can cause nausea and vomiting up to 72 hours after receiving the drug, it is essential that a patient use the prescribed antiemetic regimen around the clock through the 72-hour period.

39. **(c)** Headache is a common side effect of serotonin antagonists.

40. **(b)** The patient is experiencing an extrapyramidal effect from the metoclopramide (Reglan). Diphenhydramine (Benadryl) is used to alleviate extrapyramidal effects.

41. **(a)** Prochlorperazine (Compazine) is part of the phenothiazine class of antiemetics.

42. **(d)** Orthostatic hypotension is a common side effect, and patients need to be taught safety and movement strategies to minimize the effects of orthostatic hypotension.

43. (a)   Hiccoughs are a side effect common to corticosteroids.

44. (c)   Adverse reactions related to the central nervous system are more common in elderly patients who are using dronabinol (Marinol).

45. (d)   Use of alcohol is contraindicated while using hydroxyzine (Vistaril).

46. (b)   The patient is experiencing metabolic alkalosis, which is commonly caused by vomiting.

47. (a)   Promethazine (Phenergan) lowers the seizure threshold.

48. (c)   Buprenorphine hydrochloride (Buprenex) is an agonist-antagonist compound.

49. (b)   Morphine (regular release form) has an average onset of effect in 30 minutes and has a duration of effect from 3 to 7 hours.

50. (d)   Opioid analgesics commonly cause pupil constriction (miosis).

51. (b)   Monitoring of sedation level is more accurate than monitoring respiratory rate when assessing for respiratory depression.

52. (a)   Concomitant use of cimetidine (Tagamet) and an opioid analgesic results in an enhanced effect of the opioid analgesic.

53. (b)   Nonsteroidal anti-inflammatory agents decrease the antihypertensive effects of ACE inhibitors, beta blockers, and vasodilators.

54. (c)   Hypotension is not a symptom of opioid withdrawal.

55. (d)   Transit time in the gastrointestinal tract is slowed, thus increasing the potential for absorption.

56. (b)   The side effect of hypotension from opioids is induced by arteriolar vasodilation.

57. (c)   Muscle twitching should be reported so that further assessment can be made regarding its cause.

58. (a)   Respiratory depression is not a common problem with chronic pain.

59. (a)   Usually respiratory depression is a complication of psychotropic drugs, not hyperventilation.

60. (c)   Chinese patients may require a lower dose of benzodiazepines than usually prescribed.

61. (d)   Barbiturate toxicity manifests with hypotension; cold, clammy skin; nausea and vomiting; delirium; and generalized weakness.

62. (a)   Flurazepam is a long-acting hypnotic that commonly causes carryover effects of sedation into the daytime.

63. (b)   Liver disease is a risk factor for more adverse effects to be experienced by a patient taking triazolam (Halcion). It is important to monitor liver function tests.

64. **(a)**   Orthostatic hypotension is a common adverse effect, thus patients need to be taught safety issues related to preventing falls.

65. **(d)**   Chlordiazepoxide (Librium) is the drug of choice to treat withdrawal symptoms from alcohol. This medication also treats anxiety.

66. **(b)**   Extrapyramidal effects are common to the phenothiazine class of anti-anxiety drugs.

67. **(c)**   Fluphenazine may discolor a patient's urine to a pink or maroon color.

68. **(a)**   Haloperidol (Haldol) lowers the threshold for seizure activity. Other anti-anxiety agents should be prescribed.

69. **(d)**   Younger persons are at higher risk for depression. Also, diagnosis of a more advanced disease state is a risk factor for depression.

70. **(b)**   Anticholinergic effects, such as mouth dryness, are common with amitriptyline (Elavil). The dryness may diminish with therapy. Fluids and sugarless candy may be helpful.

71. **(a)**   Trazodone (Desyrel) belongs to the triazolopyridine class of antidepressants.

72. **(b)**   Hepatic failure can occur with the use of valproate or valproic acid (Depakote).

73. **(d)**   Carbamazepine (Tegretol) can cause leukopenia and thrombocytopenia.

74. **(c)**   Bone pain is common to both sargramostin (Leukine) and to filgrastim (Neupogen).

75. **(a)**   Hypertension is a common adverse reaction with erythropoietin (Procrit). A patient with uncontrolled hypertension may not be a candidate for the therapy.

76. **(b)**   Diabetes may be exacerbated by the use of growth factors.

*77. **(a)**   Risk factors for infections from altered phagocytic defenses include granulocyte count less than $1000/mm^3$, use of steroids, previous antibiotic therapy, diabetes, and renal disease.

*78. **(c)**   First generation cephalosporins, which include cephalothin (Keflin), cause a cross sensitivity in 5% to 15% of individuals with allergies to penicillin G.

*79. **(a)**   Vancomycin can cause phlebitis, ototoxicity, vertigo, and dizziness. If the drug were used in this patient, it would be difficult to distinguish side effects from the drug from signs and symptoms of the patient's medical condition.

*80. **(d)**   Dexamethasone (Decadron) is a long-acting corticosteroid.

*81. **(b)**   Naproxen (Naprosyn) can cause fluid retention.

*82. **(a)**   Phenytoin (Dilantin) suspension has erratic absorption.

*83. **(c)**   If the systolic blood pressure falls more than 20 mm Hg, the drug should be held and the physician notified.

*84. **(a)**   Orthostatic hypotension is an adverse reaction to dronabinol (Marinol).

* Reflects advanced oncology nursing content

PROTECTIVE MECHANISMS

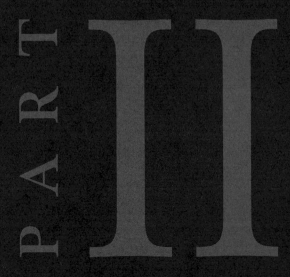

CHAPTER 11

Alterations in Mobility, Skin Integrity, and Neurologic Status

QUESTIONS

1. A patient with a brain tumor is experiencing an unsteady gait with fine hand tremors. This altered mobility may be caused by a problem in the:
   a. Limbic system.
   b. Thalamus.
   c. Cerebellum.
   d. Pons.

2. Physical examination of an adult cancer patient reveals a positive Babinski sign. How did the patient react when the lateral aspect of the sole of the foot was stroked?
   a. The toes contracted and were drawn together.
   b. The toes fanned out and were drawn back.
   c. The foot dorsiflexed with no contraction of the toes.
   d. Plantar flexion occurred with no response noted in the toes.

3. Cancer treatments associated with causing mobility problems include all of the following EXCEPT:
   a. Corticosteroids.
   b. Biotherapy.
   c. Radiation.
   d. Chemotherapy.

4. Assisting a patient with mobility impairment to achieve independence is best accomplished when the nurse:
   a. Provides reinforcement of success attained.
   b. Develops long-term outcomes for the patient.
   c. Notes problems in the patient's performance.
   d. Shows the patient methods to attain independence.

5. All of the following are methods to maximize patient safety EXCEPT:
   a. Keep floors clear of objects and debris.
   b. Keep the bed in the lowest position.
   c. Always check bath water with an elbow.
   d. Always keep side rails up.

6. A potentially serious skin disorder associated with cancer treatment is:
   a. Leukoplakia.
   b. Actinic keratosis.
   c. Mycosis fungoides.
   d. Graft versus host disease.

7. Physical examination of a 70-year-old lung cancer patient reveals thin, fragile, bruised skin on the arms and legs. The skin also has poor turgor. Which of the following treatments is most likely the cause of these findings?
   a. Radiation therapy.
   b. Steroid therapy.
   c. Antibiotic therapy.
   d. Chemotherapy.

8. An appropriate nursing intervention to minimize the risk of skin problems includes instructing a patient to:
   a. Use over-the-counter steroid creams to provide skin lubrication.
   b. Assess the skin every 48 hours.
   c. Avoid staying in one position longer than 2 hours.
   d. Massage all areas of the body to improve circulation.

9. A patient receiving vincristine (Oncovin) therapy says to the nurse, "I just can't seem to walk right. My feet feel like pins and needles." The patient is most likely experiencing:
   a. Peripheral neuropathy.
   b. Spinal cord compression.
   c. Nephrotoxicity.
   d. Peripheral myopathy.

10. Risk for constipation is listed on a care plan for a patient with neuropathy. What daily measures are needed to minimize constipation?
    a. Stool softeners.
    b. Digital rectal examination.
    c. Saline laxatives.
    d. Mineral oil lubricants.

11. Care of a patient with peripheral neuropathy includes patient education regarding:
    a. The use of oxycodone for pain control for the neuropathies.
    b. The use of counter-stimulation to minimize the paresthesia.
    c. The use of gloves to protect hands.
    d. The need to ambulate independently daily to prevent muscle dysfunction.

12. Which of the following tests is used to evaluate neuropathy?
    a. Magnetic resonance imaging.
    b. Electromyography.
    c. Myelogram.
    d. Lumbar puncture.

13. Within 24 hours of completing his initial chemotherapy treatment, a patient with lung cancer begins to experience labile emotions with slurred speech. The cause for these findings may be:
    a. Carboplatin (Paraplatin).
    b. Cyclophosphamide (Cytoxan).
    c. Etoposide (VP-16).
    d. Ifosfamide (Ifex).

14. Which of the following nursing interventions is appropriate for a patient experiencing altered thought processes?
    a. Communicate using simple terms.
    b. Allow the patient to make decisions.
    c. Keep the patient's environment unstructured.
    d. Reorient thoughts only as needed.

15. Altered sexuality may result from face and jaw neuropathy in a patient treated for head and neck cancer. What nursing interventions can be suggested to assist the patient in dealing with this?
    a. Encourage kissing to improve feelings of sexuality.
    b. Suggest other methods to express affection.
    c. Refer to a counselor to deal with sexual issues.
    d. Inform the patient the neuropathy is temporary.

*16. Which of the following assessment tests would indicate cerebellar dysfunction?
a. Positive Romberg's sign.
b. Positive Schilling test.
c. Positive Murphy's sign.
d. Positive Kernig's sign.

*17. While receiving sulfisoxazole for a urinary infection, Ms. Jenkins experienced scattered, tender subcutaneous nodules in the anterior aspect of her legs. This condition is known as:
a. Erythema multiforme.
b. Seborrheic dermatitis.
c. Erythema nodosum.
d. Pemphigus vulgaris.

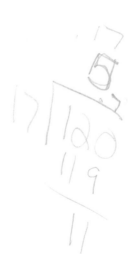

ANSWERS

1. **(c)** The cerebellum coordinates body movement.

2. **(b)** Alteration of the central nervous system in the adult can be assessed by a positive Babinski sign, in which a patient's toes fan out and are drawn back after the lateral aspect of the sole of the foot is stroked.

3. **(b)** Biotherapy is usually not associated with causing mobility problems.

4. **(a)** Providing positive reinforcement for tasks accomplished contributes to outcome achievement.

5. **(c)** Bath water is best measured using a thermometer.

6. **(d)** Graft versus host disease is a skin disorder that can occur after bone marrow transplant.

7. **(b)** Steroid therapy often results in fragile, thin, ecchymotic skin.

8. **(c)** To prevent skin breakdown or ulceration, it is imperative that patients do not stay in one position for longer than 2 hours.

9. **(a)** Vincristine (Oncovin) often causes peripheral neuropathy.

10. **(a)** Stool softeners are a safe and effective way to minimize constipation.

11. **(c)** With diminished sensation to the hands, an important intervention is to wear gloves to protect the hands from injury.

12. **(b)** An electromyogram identifies nerve degeneration and muscle atrophy related to neuropathy.

13. **(d)** Ifosfamide (Ifex) can cause confusion, hallucinations, and disorientation.

14. **(a)** Using simple terms and concise language facilitates cognitive function.

15. **(b)** Helping the patient to learn other ways of sexual expression is most appropriate.

*16. **(a)** A cerebellar dysfunction is indicated by a positive Romberg's sign.

*17. **(c)** A hypersensitivity reaction to sulfonamides that results in subcutaneous nodules that are tender and located on the anterior portion of the legs is known as erythema nodosum.

---

* Reflects advanced oncology nursing content

12

Myelosuppression

QUESTIONS

1. After 4 days of treatment with a broad spectrum cephalosporin, a patient with kidney cancer continues to experience fevers of 100.5° F to 101.2° F daily. What agent should be added to the regimen?
    a. A colony-stimulating factor.
    b. A penicillin-based antibiotic.
    c. An aminoglycoside.
    d. An antifungal.

2. Granulocyte colony-stimulating factor (Filgastrim, Neupogen) is administered for up to 14 days or until:
    a. The absolute neutrophil count is at 5000/mm^3.
    b. The absolute neutrophil count is greater than 10,000/mm^3.
    c. The patient experiences bone pain.
    d. The symptoms of febrile neutropenia are gone.

3. The most common presenting sign of infection in a patient with neutropenia is:
    a. Fever.
    b. Redness at a venous access device site.
    c. Positive blood culture.
    d. Dyspnea.

4. Five days after receiving chemotherapy, a patient presents to the clinic with a white blood cell count of 2500/mm^3 with 12% segs and 15% bands. What is the patient's absolute granulocyte count?
    a. 300/mm^3.
    b. 375/mm^3.
    c. 675/mm^3.
    d. 925/mm^3.

5. A patient with leukemia has developed neutropenia with a white blood cell count of 1200/mm^3. Which of the following statements indicates patient understanding of minimizing infection?
    a. "I should eat as many fresh fruits and vegetables as I can to keep my nutrition at a high level."
    b. "I need to monitor my temperature daily and call the doctor if it's over 102° F.
    c. "I need to get my immunizations up to date to prevent illness such as influenza."
    d. "I will avoid people who have illnesses, especially colds."

6. Upon hearing the news that he will need to give a stool sample, a cancer patient receiving chemotherapy protests, stating, "My disease isn't down there, why do you need a sample of my stool?" The nurse's best response is:
    a. "Many infections in chemotherapy patients start in the gastrointestinal tract, so it's important to monitor this."
    b. "This is a routine test used to assess for complications from chemotherapy."
    c. "Only *E. coli* bacteria can cause serious infection in the gastrointestinal tract, and it's important it's monitored.
    d. "In order to prevent infection, it's essential to find the sources of bacteria."

7. Endotoxins released from microbes during an infection predispose a cancer patient to:
    a. Pulmonary edema.
    b. Altered platelet function.
    c. Lowered red blood cell count.
    d. Hypoglycemia.

8. Mr. Smith, a newly diagnosed lymphoma patient, arrives at the clinic with a platelet count of 17,000/mm^3. What blood product should be administered?
   a. Cryoprecipitate.
   b. Random donor platelets.
   c. Human leukocyte antigen–matched platelets.
   d. Fresh frozen plasma.

9. Thrombopoietin treats thrombocytopenia by:
   a. Diminishing the destruction of platelets.
   b. Improving the function of platelets.
   c. Promoting the maturation of megakarocytes.
   d. Maintaining the quantity of matured platelets.

10. A patient with a platelet count of 50,000/mm^3 should be advised that:
    a. Spontaneous bleeding may occur.
    b. Trauma will increase the risk of bleeding.
    c. Serious bleeding of the GI tract is possible.
    d. Scleral hemorrhages will occur.

11. On the nurse's initial shift assessment, she notes the patient is lethargic, somewhat confused, and has petechiae on his feet and calves. When checking his lab work, his platelet count is 5000/mm^3. The patient's clinical state suggests:
    a. Brain herniation.
    b. Disseminated intravascular coagulation.
    c. Alveolar hemorrhage.
    d. Intracranial bleeding.

12. In treating a patient with nosebleeds related to thrombocytopenia, it is important to place the patient in which position?
    a. High Fowler's.
    b. Semi-Fowler's.
    c. Lateral.
    d. Head and neck hyperextended.

13. Which malignancy serves as a higher risk factor for the development of infection?
    a. Hepatocellular cancer.
    b. Prostate cancer.
    c. Acute lymphoblastic leukemia.
    d. Sarcoma.

14. While caring for a hospitalized cancer patient at risk for infection, it is important the nurse do which of the following?
    a. Assess vital signs every 8 hours.
    b. Perform an assessment of body systems every 4 to 8 hours.
    c. Maintain intravenous hydration to prevent dehydration.
    d. Assess blood counts every 12 hours.

15. A patient going home after induction chemotherapy for acute myelogenous leukemia should receive instruction about which of the following self-care interventions?
    a. Always wash hands after using the toilet.
    b. Take a bath or shower every other day.
    c. Perform oral care every 4 hours.
    d. If needed, administer glycerin suppositories to prevent constipation.

16. Of the following leukemias, which has a propensity to cause hemorrhage?
- a. Hairy cell leukemia.
- b. Chronic myelocytic leukemia.
- c. Acute lymphocytic leukemia.
- d. Promyelocytic leukemia.

17. Early treatment of a patient who is bleeding includes the administration of:
- a. Intravenous fluids.
- b. Vasopressor drugs.
- c. Corticosteroids.
- d. Protamine sulfate.

18. A patient with pancreatic cancer is experiencing severe shivering with fever. In addition to acetaminophen, the nurse can expect to administer:
- a. Meperidine (Demerol).
- b. Morphine.
- c. Alprazalom (Xanax).
- d. Oxazepam (Serax).

19. Which of the following is important to teach a patient at risk for developing fever?
- a. Take alcohol baths.
- b. Increase clothing layers.
- c. Remove damp clothing.
- d. Take warm sponge baths.

20. Consequences of prolonged fever include all of the following EXCEPT:
- a. Muscle weakness.
- b. Nausea.
- c. Fatigue.
- d. Myalgia.

*21. Many risk factors exist for thrombocytopenia in cancer patients. Which of the following is a condition that can lead to hypercoagulation-induced thrombocytopenia?
- a. Multiple myeloma.
- b. Liver disease.
- c. Vitamin K deficiency.
- d. Paraneoplastic syndrome.

*22. A patient with prostate cancer has become agitated. The nurse's assessment reveals petechiae on the feet, hypotension, and oozing of blood on the patient's IV dressing. Blood for lab work was drawn, with results showing: Hgb, 8.9 g/dL; Plts, 48,000/mm^3; PT, 30 seconds; PTT, 64 seconds; fibrogen, 100 mg/dL. Which of the following blood components should be administered to the patient first?
- a. Cryoprecipitate.
- b. Platelets.
- c. Fresh frozen plasma.
- d. Packed red blood cells.

---

* Reflects advanced oncology nursing content

Answers

1. **(d)**   If a patient has been on antibiotics for 3 days and fever continues, an antifungal is usually initiated next.

2. **(b)**   Granulocyte colony-stimulating factor is administered for up to 2 weeks or until the absolute neutrophil count is greater than $10,000/mm^3$.

3. **(a)**   Fever may be the only sign of infection in a patient with neutropenia, since the quantity and quality of phagocytic cells is diminished. Thus, redness and inflammatory responses may not occur.

4. **(c)**   The absolute granulocyte count is $675/mm^3$.

5. **(d)**   It is important to avoid people with communicable diseases.

6. **(a)**   Since up to 85% of infections in the cancer patient can arise from microbes in the gastrointestinal and respiratory tracts, culture of those areas helps to provide information about sources of infection.

7. **(b)**   Endotoxins released during an infectious process can damage platelets and alter platelet function.

8. **(b)**   Random donor platelets would be an appropriate choice for this patient, since he is newly diagnosed.

9. **(c)**   Thrombopoietin promotes the production and maturation of megakarocytes.

10. **(b)**   Platelet counts between $40,000/mm^3$ and $60,000/mm^3$ are associated with an increased risk of bleeding from trauma and following surgical procedures.

11. **(d)**   The patient's clinical signs indicate intracranial bleeding.

12. **(a)**   A high Fowler's position is the safest position for a patient experiencing a nosebleed.

13. **(c)**   Hematologic and lymphoid malignancies are more often associated with infection than other malignancies.

14. **(b)**   The assessment of body systems every 4 to 8 hours will facilitate early detection of signs of infection.

15. **(c)**   Meticulous personal hygiene, including skin care, perineal care, and oral care, is essential to minimize infection.

16. **(d)**   Promyelocytic leukemia is associated with bleeding.

17. **(a)**   Intravenous fluids are an initial treatment in the patient with hemorrhage.

18. **(a)**   Meperidine is effective in treating shivering chills.

19. **(c)**   By removing damp clothing, the risk of chilling is diminished.

20. **(b)**   Nausea is not a usual consequence of prolonged fever.

*21. (d)   Paraneoplastic syndrome as well as disseminated intravascular coagulation are conditions that lead to hypercoagulation-induced thrombocytopenia.

*22. (c)   The patient's clinical signs and lab work indicate disseminated intravascular coagulation. Fresh frozen plasma will assist in replacing the clotting factors.

GASTRO-INTESTINAL AND URINARY FUNCTION

PART III

CHAPTER 13

Alterations in Nutrition

QUESTIONS

1. Which of the following is not a causative factor of anorexia?
   a. Liver failure.
   b. Adverse effects of medications.
   c. Renal dysfunction.
   d. Side effects of cancer treatment.

2. Which of the following lab values would correspond to a patient experiencing anorexia?
   a. Decreased serum albumin.
   b. Increased serum transferrin.
   c. Increased total protein.
   d. Normal lymphocyte count.

3. A lung cancer patient admitted to your unit is experiencing anorexia. He states "I don't have any appetite, so why eat?" What is the best method to gather dietary information about the patient?
   a. A diet plan.
   b. A calorie count.
   c. A food diary.
   d. 24-hour food recall.

4. In planning outcomes for a patient with anorexia, it is important that the patient identify conditions in which professional assistance is needed, such as when:
   a. Nausea and vomiting are intermittent.
   b. Weight loss of more than 1 pound per day occurs.
   c. Taste abnormalities occur daily.
   d. Dyspnea is present.

5. Nutritional education for a patient with anorexia would include:
   a. Add nonfat dry milk powder to foods.
   b. Consume three meals a day.
   c. Increase the use of green leafy vegetables.
   d. Increase liquids at meals.

6. Which of the following medications is best suited to stimulate appetite in a patient with anorexia?
   a. Metoclopramide (Reglan).
   b. Megestrol acetate (Megace).
   c. Dronabinol (Marinol).
   d. Prochlorperazine (Compazine).

7. A home health nurse examines a patient with colon cancer and finds a wasting appearance, no body fat stores, and weight loss of 10 pounds in 1 week. The nurse suspects the patient has signs and symptoms of:
   a. Hemodilution.
   b. Dehydration.
   c. Malnutrition.
   d. Infection.

8. A family member is caring for a bed bound hospice patient. In teaching the caregiver about the patient's food intake, it is important to:
   a. Encourage intake but not force the patient to eat.
   b. Always use dietary supplements.
   c. Monitor the patient's weight daily.
   d. Increase the patient's intake of fruits and vegetables.

9. A patient with dysphagia is experiencing a high fever, coughing, and midchest discomfort. These findings suggest:
   a. Sepsis.
   b. Aspiration pneumonia.
   c. Congestive heart failure.
   d. Airway obstruction.

10. Which of the following malignancies is most related to the incidence of dysphagia?
    a. Primary stomach cancer.
    b. Metastatic colon cancer.
    c. Primary brain cancer.
    d. Metastatic lung cancer.

11. All of the following can be causes of dysphagia in the patient with cancer EXCEPT:
    a. Surgical resection.
    b. Radiation fibrosis.
    c. Candidiasis.
    d. Opioid analgesics.

12. In using thickening agents for patients with dysphagia, it is important to note that the greatest amount of coordination is needed for swallowing:
    a. Liquids of thin consistency.
    b. Liquids of thick consistency.
    c. Soft foods.
    d. Solid foods.

13. The nurse suggests a referral to which of the following for prolonged dysphagia?
    a. Ear, nose, and throat specialist.
    b. Speech therapist.
    c. Respiratory therapist.
    d. Oral surgeon.

14. Mrs. Jones complains that "food seems to get stuck in my throat" and "I seem to drool a lot." How can the nurse best assist her?
    a. Instruct the patient to use a long-handled spoon to place food further back in the mouth.
    b. Cut up the patient's food in small chunks.
    c. Provide an ample amount of liquid to help food pass down the esophagus.
    d. Instruct the patient to tilt her head back to help her swallowing reflex.

15. A treatment of choice for long-term nutritional management of dysphagia in a patient with head and neck cancer is:
    a. Peripheral supplemental nutrition.
    b. Nasogastric tube feeding.
    c. Feeding via a percutaneous gastrostomy.
    d. Total parenteral nutrition.

16. Xerostomia is characterized by:
    a. Inflammation of the salivary glands.
    b. A decrease in the production of saliva.
    c. Oral lesions.
    d. Leukoplakia.

17. Which of the following statements by a throat cancer patient undergoing radiation indicates the need for further teaching?
    a. "I'll need to start drinking decaffeinated coffee."
    b. "Since I have cancer there's no need to stop smoking now."
    c. "I'll need to stop having my after-dinner cocktail."
    d. "Moist foods will work better with my treatment."

18. A drug of choice to increase the flow of saliva in a patient with xerostomia is:
    a. Prednisolone (Anticulose).
    b. Acetylcysteine (Mucosil).
    c. Saliva substitute (Salivart).
    d. Pilocarpine (Salagen).

19. To enhance the moisture of the oral cavity, a patient can be advised to:
    a. Use a room humidifier.
    b. Minimize daily tooth brushing.
    c. Rinse frequently with a commercial mouthwash.
    d. Suck on peppermint candy.

20. A patient states, "I use meat tenderizer before I eat to help with my mouth dryness." The nurse understands this is an acceptable treatment because:
    a. The substance coats the oral mucosa.
    b. The substance breaks up thick saliva.
    c. The substance protects the oral cavity.
    d. The substance minimizes mucosal irritation.

21. A patient with Hodgkin's disease has just completed midchest radiation therapy. The patient reports odynophagia and epigastric pain. The nurse suspects the patient has developed:
    a. Hypogeusia.
    b. Stomatitis.
    c. Esophagitis.
    d. Enteritis.

22. Mucositis is more likely to occur in which of the following malignant conditions?
    a. Melanoma.
    b. Leukemia.
    c. Breast cancer.
    d. Prostate cancer.

23. After completing radiation therapy, a patient experiences jaw pain and spasms. The nurse informs the patient that this condition can be related to mucositis and is called:
    a. Odontitis.
    b. Ageusia.
    c. Osteonecrosis.
    d. Trismus.

24. Which of the following is not considered a risk factor for stomatitis?
    a. Periodontal disease.
    b. Poor fitting dentures.
    c. Older age.
    d. Dehydration.

25. Which of the following patients is at greater risk for developing stomatitis?
    a. A patient receiving a 5-day continuous infusion of 5-fluorouracil (5-Fu) for a total treatment of 6 months.
    b. A patient receiving nitrogen mustard (Mustargen) per IV bolus once every 2 weeks for 8 months.
    c. A patient receiving hydroxyurea (Hydrea) for 30 days.
    d. A patient receiving vinorelbine (Navelbine) by IV bolus once every week for 6 months.

26. When examining a patient's mouth, the nurse notes isolated white patches and oral lesions. The nurse knows this finding equates with which classification of oral mucositis?
    a. Grade 1.
    b. Grade 2.
    c. Grade 3.
    d. Grade 4.

27. A patient completed doxorubicin (Adriamycin) treatment 1 week ago. Today the patient is experiencing a stinging sensation in the mouth. The nurse asks the patient to watch for what over the next 3 to 5 days?
    a. Oral sores.
    b. Mouth dryness.
    c. Taste changes.
    d. Cracked lips.

28. Which of the following measures is least effective in minimizing stomatitis?
    a. Encourage frequent oral hygiene.
    b. Encourage fluid intake of 2000 mL or more.
    c. Avoid spicy and citrus-based foods.
    d. Encourage hot tea with honey to soothe oral lesions.

29. A patient with grade 1 stomatitis asks his nurse what type of mouth solution he should use. The nurse responds by suggesting the patient use:
    a. Cepacol mouthwash.
    b. Saline solution.
    c. Hydrogen peroxide (full strength).
    d. Chlorhexidine solution.

30. Chemotherapy-induced taste alterations often result in:
    a. Increased threshold for bitter taste.
    b. Aversion to fats.
    c. Metallic taste sensations.
    d. Decreased threshold for salty tastes.

31. Which of the following nutritional deficiencies is associated with taste alterations?
    a. Zinc.
    b. Potassium.
    c. Vitamin E.
    d. Sodium.

32. Consequences of taste changes include all of the following EXCEPT:
   a. Weight loss.
   b. Anorexia.
   c. Excess saliva.
   d. Protein loss.

33. A nurse may suggest to a patient with taste aversions to:
   a. Avoid sauces or gravies on foods.
   b. Add large amounts of seasonings to enhance food flavors.
   c. Marinate meats to enhance or disguise flavor.
   d. Decrease fluid intake with meal.

34. Causes of nausea in the cancer patient include all of the following EXCEPT:
   a. Cancer treatment.
   b. Food toxins.
   c. Anxiety.
   d. Increased gastric emptying.

35. A patient with prolonged nausea may experience which of the following?
   a. Hypermagnesemia.
   b. Hypokalemia.
   c. Hypernatremia.
   d. Hypocalcemia.

36. A patient tells her nurse, "I can't stand to take these antinausea pills anymore! There must be something else I can do to beat this nausea." The nurse suggests a behavioral intervention such as:
   a. Guided imagery.
   b. Acupuncture.
   c. Transcutaneous electrical nerve stimulation.
   d. Discussion therapy.

37. Symptoms of nausea include:
   a. Diaphoresis and bradycardia.
   b. Dizziness and decreased salivation.
   c. Diaphoresis and tachycardia.
   d. Dizziness and bradycardia.

38. To prevent dehydration in a patient with nausea, the nurse suggests the following:
   a. Drink warm broth.
   b. Eat ice pops.
   c. Drink milk shakes.
   d. Eat yogurt.

39. A patient with a brain tumor has just received her first IV dose of 100 mg of carmustine (BCNU). She was premedicated with 30 mg ondansetron (Zofran) IV and 20 mg of dexamethasone (Decadron). She's going home with 30-mg prochlorperazine (Compazine) spansules. The nurse instructs the patient as follows:
   a. "Wait at least 8 hours before starting this medication."
   b. "Use this medication only if you feel nauseated."
   c. "Take your antinausea medication as prescribed every 4 to 6 hours for the next 48 hours."
   d. "Do not eat for the next 24 hours to prevent nausea."

40. A chemotherapy patient immediately vomits each week on entering the treatment room. The patient asks, "Why does this happen? I feel fine until I get here." The best response the nurse can give is:
    a. "Don't be concerned about it. We expect this response in patients."
    b. "Eating a light snack before coming to your chemo appointment will help."
    c. "About one fourth of chemotherapy patients have anticipatory vomiting, which is a conditioned response."
    d. "Keeping your stomach empty will decrease your chance of vomiting."

41. Which nursing diagnosis is least related to a patient experiencing vomiting?
    a. Skin integrity impairment.
    b. Fluid volume deficit.
    c. Fatigue.
    d. Altered nutrition, less than body requirements.

42. A patient receiving abdominal radiation for advanced colon cancer has been experiencing intermittent vomiting for the past 7 days, despite using his antiemetic. His weight has dropped from 165 pounds to 150 pounds. He is pale, with poor skin turgor and dark urine. The patient should:
    a. Increase his dose of antiemetic medication.
    b. Phone his physician.
    c. Ingest clear fluids to 2000 mL/day.
    d. Keep his environment cool and humidified.

43. A patient with breast cancer confides in the nurse that she has gained weight since starting treatment with tamoxifen citrate (Nolvadex). The patient asks why she is gaining weight. The nurse responds:
    a. "You need to increase your activity level."
    b. "You're electrolytes are not within normal limits, so that's why you're gaining weight."
    c. "A potential side effect of your drug treatment is weight gain."
    d. "You do need to watch your total caloric intake while undergoing cancer treatment."

44. Weight loss in a cancer patient can be the result of:
    a. Draining wounds.
    b. Steroids.
    c. Hypernatremia.
    d. Hypoglycemia.

45. A nurse is contacted by a patient with liver cancer who states, "I eat some food every day, but I keep losing weight, can you help me?" The nurse offers the following suggestion:
    a. Increase the percentage of carbohydrate foods to provide glucose for calories and energy.
    b. Plan four meals per day that are high in proteins and vitamins.
    c. Eat high-calorie, high-protein foods when the appetite is strongest.
    d. Ingest full strength dietary liquid supplements at least four times per day.

46. Skin changes may be indicative of nutritional disturbances. Which of the following is least connected to poor nutrition?
    a. Bleeding gums.
    b. Brittle nails.
    c. Skin ulcers.
    d. Flaky skin.

47. Cachexia is defined as:
  a. Loss of appetite.
  b. A syndrome of progressive wasting.
  c. A syndrome of nutrients supporting tumor growth.
  d. Anemia accompanied by weight loss.

48. Risk factors for the development of cachexia include all of the following EXCEPT:
  a. Abdominal surgery.
  b. Chemotherapy.
  c. Depression.
  d. Ketoacidosis.

49. Which of the following is a pharmacologic intervention to stimulate appetite in cachexia?
  a. Lorazepam (Ativan).
  b. Mepromate (Equanil).
  c. Dexamethasone (Decadron).
  d. Methyldopa (Aldomet).

50. Evaluating visceral protein stores in a patient equates to assessing which lab value?
  a. Total iron-binding capacity.
  b. Hemoglobin.
  c. Serum sodium.
  d. Creatinine clearance.

51. A patient with endometrial cancer has increased abdominal girth, weight gain, dyspnea, and lower extremity edema. The patient is experiencing:
  a. Edema related to pleural effusion.
  b. Congestive heart failure related to cardiac insufficiency.
  c. Ascites related to compromised peritoneal drainage.
  d. Abdominal distention related to bowel obstruction.

52. Patient education regarding ascites should include:
  a. Use of oxygen therapy.
  b. Elevation of lower extremities.
  c. Fluid restriction instructions.
  d. Methods to perform postural drainage.

*53. A patient with metastatic bladder cancer has lost 20 pounds from his 170-pound weight 6 weeks ago. He appears pale and weak. An expected lab finding is:
  a. Pre-albumin, 22 mg/dL.
  b. Total protein, 6.0 g/dL.
  c. Total lymphocyte count, 1500/mm^3.
  d. Total iron-binding capacity, 280 μg/dL.

*54. With increasing doses of radiation to the oral cavity, the patient can expect changes in saliva. It is expected that the saliva will become more:
  a. Watery.
  b. Thick.
  c. Acidic.
  d. Frothy.

---

* Reflects advanced oncology nursing content

*55. Mucositis causes major discomfort. Which of the following vitamins can be considered a topical analgesic for mucositis?
   a. Vitamin A.
   b. Vitamin C.
   c. Vitamin D.
   d. Vitamin E.

*56. A patient with a brain tumor is experiencing polyuria, polydipsia, dry mucous membranes, irritability, and a low-grade fever. Lab work is not available yet, but the nurse suspects the patient is experiencing:
   a. Hypermagnesemia.
   b. Hypomagnesemia.
   c. Hypernatremia.
   d. Hyponatremia.

*57. A patient with mesothelioma has just undergone paracentesis to alleviate ascites. To be diagnostic of ascites related to a malignant condition, the nurse knows the evaluation of the drained fluid will show:
   a. A high level of carcinoembryonic antigen.
   b. A low level of carcinoembryonic antigen.
   c. A high level of alfa fetoprotein.
   d. A low level of alfa fetoprotein.

*58. A patient with diabetes mellitus is receiving radiation treatment for a brain tumor. He has been started on 800 mg of megestrol acetate (Megace) to stimulate appetite. It is important for the nurse to teach the patient to monitor for:
   a. Hyperglycemia and edema.
   b. Hypoglycemia and pruritis.
   c. Hypocalcemia and diaphoresis.
   d. Hypotension and photosensitivity.

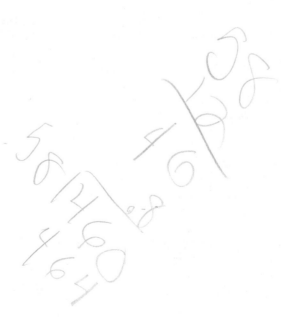

ANSWERS

1. **(c)**   Renal dysfunction is usually not a causative factor of anorexia.

2. **(a)**   Patients with anorexia experience hypoalbuminemia.

3. **(d)**   The best method at this time to gather dietary information about the patient is with a 24-hour food recall. With recalling food intake in the last 24 hours, the nurse can begin to assess eating habits.

4. **(b)**   Professional intervention is imperative if a patient with anorexia experiences weight loss of more than 1 pound per day.

5. **(a)**   The calories and protein content of food can be increased by adding nonfat dry milk to various foods.

6. **(b)**   Megestrol acetate (Megace) is used for the treatment of anorexia and weight loss.

7. **(c)**   The listed signs and symptoms are indicative of malnutrition.

8. **(a)**   Forcing a patient to eat can become counterproductive.

9. **(b)**   Aspiration and aspiration pneumonia are common consequences of dysphagia. Aspiration pneumonia is characterized by coughing, gagging, fever, and chest pain.

10. **(d)**   Individuals with metastatic lung cancer, head and neck cancer, and esophageal cancer are at an increased risk of dysphagia.

11. **(d)**   Opioid analgesics are not a causative factor of dysphagia.

12. **(a)**   Liquids of thin consistency are harder to control with dysphagia and can cause aspiration.

13. **(b)**   Speech therapists evaluate and intervene with patients experiencing swallowing problems.

14. **(a)**   Moving food from the front of the mouth to the back of the mouth may facilitate swallowing with less of a sensation of "getting stuck."

15. **(c)**   Feeding by using a dietary supplement via a percutaneous gastrostomy tube is the least invasive method with less complications for long-term use.

16. **(b)**   Xerostomia is excessive dryness of the oral cavity caused by a decreased production of saliva.

17. **(b)**   Nicotine aggravates mouth dryness.

18. **(d)**   Pilocarpine (Salagen) stimulates cholinergic receptors, resulting in the production of saliva.

19. **(a)**   A room humidifier will help provide moisture to the oral mucosa. Sugared candies and commercial mouthwashes should be avoided. Fluoride toothpaste is also important.

20. **(b)**   Meat tenderizers assist in breaking up thick saliva.

21. **(c)**   Esophagitis is mucositis of the esophagus. Esophagitis is a common side effect of chest radiation producing symptoms such as dysphagia, odynophagia, and epigastric pain.

22. **(b)**   Mucositis is two to three times more likely to occur in hematologic malignancies than solid tumors.

23. **(d)**   Trismus is caused by fibrosis of the chewing muscles and is characterized by jaw pain and spasms.

24. **(c)**   Older individuals have less frequency of stomatitis than younger individuals.

25. **(a)**   The antimetabolite class of chemotherapeutic agents is highly associated with stomatitis. Also, continuous infusion schedules cause a greater incidence of stomatitis.

26. **(b)**   Grade 2 mucositis is associated with isolated white patches and oral ulcerations.

27. **(a)**   Pain and burning can precede objective signs of mucositis, such as oral sores. Mucositis can develop within 2 weeks of chemotherapy.

28. **(d)**   Hot liquids can be irritating to the oral mucosa.

29. **(b)**   Saline solution is an effective cleansing agent for grade 1 stomatitis.

30. **(c)**   Often patients report metallic taste sensations after receiving chemotherapy.

31. **(a)**   Zinc deficiency is associated with taste alterations.

32. **(c)**   Saliva is often decreased in patients with taste changes.

33. **(c)**   The marination of meat helps to enhance the flavor or disguise the flavor of the meat.

34. **(d)**   Delayed gastric emptying usually causes nausea.

35. **(b)**   A common electrolyte imbalance that may occur in a patient dealing with prolonged nausea is hypokalemia.

36. **(a)**   Guided imagery is a behavioral intervention that may ease nausea.

37. **(c)**   Symptoms of nausea include diaphoresis, tachycardia, pallor, excessive salivation, increased weakness, and dizziness.

38. **(b)**   Ice pops provide a method to replace fluids, while minimizing the feeling of nausea.

39. **(c)**   It is important that the patient begin taking an antiemetic and continue taking the antiemetic around the clock for the best prevention of nausea.

40. **(c)**   Anticipatory nausea is a conditioned response that can be caused by poor nausea control or other noxious stimuli.

41. **(a)**   Skin integrity impairment is least related to a patient experiencing vomiting.

42. **(b)**   The patient is experiencing dehydration and a weight change of approximately 10%. A physician needs to be notified for treatment.

43. (c) Even though other factors may be present, tamoxifen citrate (Nolvadex) can cause weight gain in patients using the drug.

44. (a) Draining wounds can contribute to weight loss due to fluid drainage. Other sources of fluid loss include fistulas, sweating, and GI suction.

45. (c) Providing high-calorie, high-protein foods when the appetite is strong will help to provide nutrients to maintain weight.

46. (d) Dry, flaky skin can be the result of many factors, such as drug therapy, environment, and genetics.

47. (b) Cachexia is a syndrome of progressive loss of muscle, fat, and body weight.

48. (d) Ketoacidosis is an alteration in nutritional metabolism, but it usually does not progress to cachexia.

49. (c) Dexamethasone and other steroids stimulate appetite and can contribute to an overall sense of euphoria.

50. (a) Total iron-binding capacity is a measure of protein stores.

51. (c) Ascites is the result of compromised peritoneal drainage, in which the fluid cannot be reabsorbed into the circulating system.

52. (b) Elevation of lower extremities assists in reducing swelling and promoting comfort.

*53. (c) A total lymphocyte count of 1500/mm^3 indicates malnutrition and altered immune system competence.

*54. (b) Symptoms related to thickness of saliva are directly proportional to the amount of radiation administered.

*55. (d) Vitamin E can be applied topically to provide analgesia for mucositis.

*56. (c) The patient is exhibiting classic signs and symptoms of hypernatremia. A risk factor for the development of hypernatremia is brain tumor.

*57. (a) A high level of carcinoembryonic antigen is diagnostic of malignancy-related ascites.

*58. (a) Side effects of megestrol acetate (Megace) include hyperglycemia and edema. A diabetic patient may use this medication but should be monitored closely.

* Reflects advanced oncology nursing content

Alterations in Elimination

QUESTIONS

1. A patient is complaining of having a sudden desire to urinate, which leads to the involuntary loss of urine. The nurse suspects the patient is experiencing:
   a. Reflex incontinence.
   b. Urge incontinence.
   c. Functional incontinence.
   d. Total incontinence.

2. The loss of bladder sensation may be caused by all of the following EXCEPT:
   a. Inflammation.
   b. Infection.
   c. Bladder distention.
   d. Tissue hyperplasia.

3. Which of the following is an anticholinergic medication used to treat urinary incontinence:
   a. Oxybutynin (Ditropan).
   b. Primidone (Mysoline).
   c. Nitrofurantoin (Macrodantin).
   d. Phenazopyridine (Pyridium).

4. A patient receiving cyclophosphamide (Cytoxan) is being evaluated for hematuria. Which of the following tests would be ordered?
   a. Specific gravity.
   b. Culture and sensitivity.
   c. Urinalysis.
   d. Viscosity.

5. Which of the following interventions should be included in a bladder training program?
   a. Maintain fluid intake between 1000 and 1200 mL/day.
   b. Establish a routine schedule for voiding.
   c. Avoid asking the patient about voiding.
   d. Teach the patient to perform pelvic muscle exercises five times per day.

6. Which group of antineoplastic agents is most associated with constipation?
   a. Antitumor antibiotics.
   b. Alkylating agents.
   c. Plant alkaloids.
   d. Antimetabolites.

7. A patient with a long-standing history of constipation is admitted to the oncology unit. The patient has nausea, vomiting, and abdominal distention with pain and cramping. The admitting nurse suspects:
   a. Fecal impaction.
   b. Ascites.
   c. Peritonitis.
   d. Bowel obstruction.

8. A patient with constipation is to be discharged home. Which of the following statements indicates the patient understands when to notify a physician about a serious change related to constipation?
   a. "If I can't hear bowel sounds, I need to call the doctor."
   b. "If I continue to have problems having a bowel movement daily, I will phone my doctor."
   c. "Cramping with my enema is dangerous, and I will stop and notify the doctor."
   d. "If I feel I am becoming dependent on my laxatives, I will let the doctor know."

9. *Clostridium difficile* can cause which type of diarrhea?
   a. Osmotic diarrhea.
   b. Motile diarrhea.
   c. Secretory diarrhea.
   d. Colloid diarrhea.

10. Which of the following drugs is least associated with the development of diarrhea?
    a. Cisplatin (Platinol).
    b. 5-Fluorouracil (5-FU).
    c. Dactinomycin (Cosmegen).
    d. Methotrexate (MTX).

11. A patient with diarrhea is experiencing skin excoriation in the rectal area. The nurse suggests the following skin care regimen:
    a. Applying a zinc oxide product to the rectal area after using a periwash on the rectum.
    b. Applying an ice pack followed by protective lotion to the rectal area.
    c. Applying a transparent, protective barrier dressing to the rectal area.
    d. Cleansing the rectal area with mild soap and water and applying an ointment barrier.

12. Physical signs of diarrhea may include hyperactive bowel sounds as well as:
    a. Hard stool in the rectum.
    b. Weight gain.
    c. Increased urinary output.
    d. Loss of urgency to defecate.

13. Which of the following is a nutritional strategy to decrease bowel motility?
    a. Serve foods at a cold temperature.
    b. Avoid alcohol.
    c. Use natural spices in food.
    d. Use liquid dietary supplements.

14. Often obstructions of the large bowel occur in the sigmoid area of the colon and are caused by all of the following EXCEPT:
    a. Diverticulitis.
    b. Volvulus.
    c. Anticholinergic drugs.
    d. Cancer.

15. Nonsurgical adhesions may cause small bowel obstruction in a patient with cancer. What can cause these adhesions?
    a. Radiation therapy.
    b. Trauma.
    c. Inguinal hernia.
    d. Chemotherapy.

16. Which of the following cancers are most associated with obstruction of the bowel?
    a. Liver cancer.
    b. Ovarian cancer.
    c. Stomach cancer.
    d. Prostate cancer.

17. A serious complication associated with bowel obstruction is:
    a. Ileus.
    b. Dehydration.
    c. Perforation.
    d. Infection.

18. An emergency room nurse notes that a patient presents with a distended abdomen, borborygmi, and pain upon palpation. In addition to intravenous fluids, the nurse expects to:
    a. Initiate total parenteral nutrition.
    b. Restrict the patient to clear liquids.
    c. Give a mineral oil enema.
    d. Insert a nasogastric tube.

19. On initial assessment of a patient with a suspected bowel obstruction, which of the following diagnostic tests would be most appropriate?
    a. Oral barium and upper GI series.
    b. Barium enema and lower GI series.
    c. Chest x-ray.
    d. Colonoscopy.

20. If a patient has a mechanical obstruction of the bowel, what type of bowel sounds are often heard proximal to the obstruction?
    a. High-pitched sounds.
    b. Low-pitched sounds.
    c. Absent sounds.
    d. Normal active sounds.

21. In caring for a patient with a nasogastric tube attached to suction, the nurse should:
    a. Use sterile technique in irrigating the tube.
    b. Give the patient ice chips to keep the mouth moist.
    c. Apply a petroleum-based lubricant to nares.
    d. Irrigate the tube with normal saline.

22. When assessing for peritonitis, the nurse should be alert for the following signs and symptoms:
    a. Back pain and hypertension.
    b. Rigid abdomen and tachycardia.
    c. Hypertension and labored breathing.
    d. Bradycardia and rigid abdomen.

23. All of the following pharmacologic agents may be used to treat a bowel obstruction EXCEPT:
    a. Smooth muscle relaxants.
    b. Antiemetics.
    c. Corticosteroids.
    d. Ganglionic blockers.

24. A home health nurse suspects a problem with a patient who has a history of bowel obstruction. Which of the following findings will prompt the nurse to contact the physician?
    a. Localized intense constant pain.
    b. Absence of bowel sounds after 1 minute of auscultation.
    c. Abdominal distention.
    d. Nausea and vomiting.

25. A patient had a bowel resection with cecostomy. Which of the following is a normal finding in relation to the cecostomy?
    a. Liquid stool drains constantly.
    b. Thick fluid to mushy stool drains constantly.
    c. Mushy stool drains at intervals.
    d. Soft stool drains at intervals.

26. Which type of bowel diversion may be performed to palliate an obstruction in a patient with terminal cancer?
    a. Proximal stoma.
    b. End stoma.
    c. Loop stoma.
    d. Double barrel stoma.

27. An ileal conduit poses a high risk for:
    a. Hydronephrosis.
    b. Polyuria.
    c. Nephrotic syndrome.
    d. Urinary tract infection.

28. A patient with bladder cancer asks the nurse to provide her with further information about patients with urinary diversions. The nurse suggests the patient contact the:
    a. Oley Foundation.
    b. United Ostomy Association.
    c. American Cancer Society.
    d. National Cancer Institute.

29. When teaching a patient about colostomy care, which patient statement indicates the need for further education?
    a. "Irrigating the colostomy will help me to have regular bowel movements at more predictable times."
    b. "I should wash the skin around the stoma with clear water and carefully dry the area."
    c. "It is important to use paste around the colostomy bag to prevent leakage."
    d. "I should empty the bag when it gets three quarters full."

30. Which of the following foods will increase a colostomy patient's fiber intake but not add to an odor problem?
    a. Rice.
    b. Beans.
    c. Cabbage.
    d. Prunes.

31. Renal dysfunction can occur with multiple myeloma. Which of the following is a causative factor?
    a. Hypocalcemia.
    b. Casts.
    c. Anemia.
    d. Hypouricemia.

32. All of the following are signs and symptoms of renal dysfunction EXCEPT:
    a. Poor skin turgor.
    b. Lethargy.
    c. Hypertension.
    d. Polyuria.

*33. To treat his colon cancer, Mr. Bonner will be undergoing surgical resection of more than 75% of his large intestine. The nurse informs him that he will likely experience frequent diarrhea. When the patient asks why the diarrhea will occur, the nurse explains it is caused by:
   a. Inflammation of the bowel.
   b. Increased intestinal motility.
   c. Fluid malabsorption syndrome.
   d. Carcinoid syndrome.

*34. Mrs. Renner is receiving 2 teaspoons of psyllium (Metamucil) tid and ducosate sodium (Co-lace) 100 mg bid. In teaching the patient about her home medications, the nurse informs Mrs. Renner that she should avoid:
   a. Calcium carbonate (Maalox).
   b. Fexofenadine (Allegra).
   c. Estradiol transderm system (Estraderm).
   d. Chloral hydrate (Aquachoral).

*35. A patient with non-Hodgkin's lymphoma has been undergoing treatment for tumor lysis syndrome. The nurse needs to monitor the patient for obstructive diuresis, which occurs when:
   a. The urine dipstick is negative for uric acid.
   b. Urine output is 1000 mL in 8 hours.
   c. Serum creatinine returns to a normal level.
   d. Urine output is more than 2000 mL in 8 hours.

---

* Reflects advanced oncology nursing content

ANSWERS

1. **(b)** Urge incontinence is characterized by a sudden and strong sensation to void. Often, involuntary passage of urine results.

2. **(d)** Tissue hyperplasia is not generally associated with loss of bladder sensation.

3. **(a)** Oxybutynin (Ditropan) is an anticholinergic used to treat urinary incontinence, frequency, and urgency.

4. **(c)** The urinalysis will evaluate presence of blood in the urine.

5. **(b)** The establishment of a routine is integral to the success of a bladder training program.

6. **(c)** Plant alkaloids, such as vinblastine and vincristine, are most associated with constipation.

7. **(d)** The patient is exhibiting signs and symptoms of a bowel obstruction. Bowel obstruction is a potential outcome of long-term constipation.

8. **(a)** Absence of bowel sounds is a serious change to report to a physician.

9. **(c)** *Clostridium difficile* causes the intestinal mucosa to secrete excessive amounts of fluid. This is termed secretory diarrhea.

10. **(a)** Cisplatin (Platinol) is least associated with causing diarrhea.

11. **(d)** Mild soap used with water inhibits bacterial growth. A protective ointment serves as a skin barrier.

12. **(a)** Hard stool may be present, causing loose stool to leak around an impaction.

13. **(b)** Alcohol is a gastrointestinal stimulant, thus avoiding its use will assist in decreasing bowel motility.

14. **(c)** Anticholinergic drugs are not often the cause of obstruction in the large intestine.

15. **(a)** Nonsurgical adhesions leading to small bowel obstruction may be caused by radiation therapy or infections.

16. **(b)** Ovarian cancer commonly causes obstruction of the bowel.

17. **(c)** Even though ileus, dehydration, and infection can occur with bowel obstruction, the most serious complication is perforation.

18. **(d)** Decompression of the abdomen via nasogastric tube is a basic component of the medical management of the patient with a suspected bowel obstruction.

19. **(b)** Barium enema is the diagnostic test used to evaluate for bowel obstruction.

20. **(a)** High-pitched, tinkling bowel sounds are often heard in the abdominal area proximal to a bowel obstruction.

21. **(d)** Irrigating with normal saline facilitates the patency of the nasogastric tube.

22. **(b)** Signs of peritonitis include rigid abdomen, increased pain, shallow respirations, and tachycardia.

23. **(d)** Ganglionic blockers may actually cause bowel obstruction.

24. **(a)** Localized intense pain may indicate a complication of a bowel obstruction.

25. **(b)** A cecostomy produces semifluid to mushy stool. Drainage occurs constantly throughout a 24-hour period.

26. **(c)** A loop stoma is a temporary procedure where a loop of bowel is brought out through an abdominal incision. This procedure is used to provide palliation for patients with obstructions.

27. **(d)** There is a high potential for the development of urinary tract infection with an ileal conduit, because the system has much reflux occurring.

28. **(b)** The United Ostomy Association is an appropriate support group for a patient to gain further information about others with urinary diversions.

29. **(d)** It is important for the patient with a colostomy to empty the bag when it is one-third to one-half full. This will prevent the pouch from disengaging and causing fecal spilling.

30. **(a)** Rice will provide roughage but does not contribute to producing gas in the gastrointestinal tract.

31. **(b)** Dense casts tend to infiltrate the renal tubules, causing obstruction and dysfunction of the kidney.

32. **(c)** Signs and symptoms of renal dysfunction include arrhythmias, orthostatic hypotension, weak pulse, lethargy, confusion, poor skin turgor, nausea and vomiting, and various genitourinary problems, such as polyuria, oliguria, and flank pain.

*33. **(c)** With the resection of a significant amount of the bowel, malabsorption of fluid occurs causing diarrhea.

*34. **(a)** Constipation is a frequent side effect of calcium carbonate (Maalox).

*35. **(d)** When an obstruction is removed within the renal system, such as the clearance of uric acid crystals in tumor lysis syndrome, obstructive diuresis may result. Obstructive diuresis is defined as urine output of more than 2000 mL in 8 hours.

---

* Reflects advanced oncology nursing content

CARDIO-PULMONARY FUNCTION

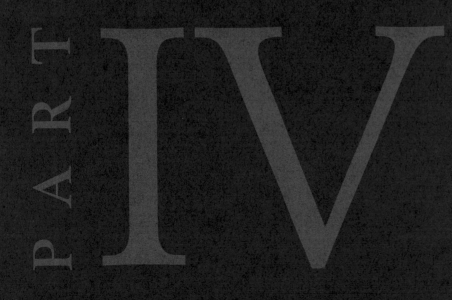

PART IV

Alterations in
Ventilation

QUESTIONS

1. When a complete pneumothorax is present, it may cause mediastinal shift. A mediastinal shift may lead to:
   a. Rupture of the pericardial sac.
   b. Decreased filling of the heart.
   c. Increased cardiac output.
   d. Rupture of the aorta.

2. An important nursing intervention to prevent laryngeal edema immediately after a bronchoscopy is to:
   a. Apply a cool-mist oxygen face tent.
   b. Provide ice chips to suck on.
   c. Provide adequate pain control.
   d. Administer lidocaine (Xylocaine) spray.

3. Immediately after a thoracentesis is completed, it is important for the nurse to assess the patient for:
   a. Decreased respiratory rate.
   b. Increased breath sounds.
   c. Expectoration of blood.
   d. Increased blood pressure.

4. An appropriate outcome for a patient with altered perfusion and ventilation is:
   a. The patient states methods to conserve energy and minimize fatigue.
   b. The patient verbalizes ways he can depend on his family to provide for his activities of daily living.
   c. The patient identifies that his prescribed oxygen is only to be used on an as-needed basis.
   d. The patient states that friends and family should only visit in the evening.

5. A patient with lung cancer is experiencing shortness of breath and tachypnea. Which of the following drugs would best treat this respiratory impairment?
   a. Meperidine (Demerol).
   b. Morphine sulfate.
   c. Hydroxyzine (Vistaril).
   d. Midazolam (Versed).

6. Radiation-induced pneumonitis is most likely to occur in a patient with:
   a. Congestive heart failure.
   b. Lobectomy.
   c. Lung tissue inflammation.
   d. Cardiovascular disease.

7. Pulmonary fibrosis results from direct injury to the:
   a. Alveolar tissue.
   b. Bronchioles.
   c. Trachea.
   d. Pleural cavity.

8. Mild symptoms related to pulmonary toxicity can be managed with:
   a. Cough suppressant therapy.
   b. Glucocorticoid therapy.
   c. Bronchodilator therapy.
   d. Diuretic therapy.

9. In preventing Bleomycin (Blenoxane)–associated pulmonary fibrosis, it is important to limit the cumulative dose to:
   a. 400 mg/m^2 or less.
   b. 400 units or less.
   c. 550 mg/m^2 or less.
   d. 550 units or less.

10. Methotrexate (MTX) is associated with pulmonary toxicity through a hypersensitivity reaction. Because of the presence of a hypersensitivity factor, it is important for the nurse to assess for:
   a. Liver complications.
   b. Pulmonary complications.
   c. Capillary leak syndrome.
   d. Renal dysfunction.

11. Two significant factors related to the development of pulmonary fibrosis from carmustine (BCNU) therapy are the total cumulative dose of more than 1500 mg/m^2 and:
   a. Oxygen therapy.
   b. Radiation therapy.
   c. Concomitant cardiac disease.
   d. Preexisting lung disease.

12. When does radiation therapy–related pulmonary toxicity usually occur?
   a. 3 weeks after starting treatment.
   b. 6 weeks after starting treatment.
   c. 2 to 3 months after completing treatment.
   d. 6 months after completing treatment.

13. On physical examination, what would be considered a late sign of radiation-induced pulmonary toxicity?
   a. Cyanosis.
   b. Pleural friction rub.
   c. Rapid, shallow respirations.
   d. Bilateral rales.

14. With regard to pulmonary toxicity caused by cancer treatment, a pulmonary function test will reveal which of the following?
   a. Increased lung volume.
   b. Decreased lung volume.
   c. Increased diffusion capacity.
   d. Decreased airway resistance.

15. In a patient experiencing dyspnea, which of the following drugs would best increase air flow to the lungs?
   a. Albuterol (Ventolin).
   b. Diazepam (Valium).
   c. Hydromorphone (Dilaudid).
   d. Acetylcysteine (Mucomyst).

16. Signs and symptoms of dyspnea include:
   a. Productive cough, nostril flaring, fever.
   b. Tachypnea, nostril flaring, digital clubbing.
   c. Productive cough, digital clubbing, wheezing.
   d. Tachypnea, wheezing, fever.

17. To minimize the sensation of dyspnea, a patient should be advised to:
    a. Perform low-impact exercises.
    b. Breathe using a rapid, shallow pattern.
    c. Maintain bedrest.
    d. Practice relaxation techniques.

18. The nurse is evaluating discharge education for a patient with dyspnea. The nurse knows the patient has an understanding of the discharge instructions when the patient states:
    a. "I will contact my doctor if I have sudden pain."
    b. "I won't worry if I have skin changes, since this does not have anything to do with my breathing."
    c. "I will make sure to continue my schedule at home, since activity is good for my breathing."
    d. "Oxygen therapy has no side effects and it will always help my breathing."

19. Malignant pleural effusion may be caused by:
    a. Increased hydrostatic pressure in the pleural space.
    b. Decreased permeability of the pleural endothelium.
    c. Increased negative pressure within the pleural space.
    d. Increased capillary permeability.

20. Common malignancies that cause pleural effusions are:
    a. Breast, lung, lymphoma.
    b. Breast, lung, prostate.
    c. Lung, brain, bone.
    d. Lymphoma, kidney, breast.

21. Which of the following is used as a sclerosing agent to treat pleural effusion?
    a. Lidocaine (Xylocaine).
    b. Methotrexate (MTX).
    c. Nitrogen mustard (Mustargen).
    d. Thiotepa (Thioplex).

22. Which of the following are the most common signs and symptoms of pleural effusion?
    a. Nonproductive cough, chest pain, dyspnea.
    b. Productive cough, chest pain, decreased cardiac output.
    c. Nonproductive cough, dyspnea, increased breath sounds.
    d. Productive cough, dyspnea, bradycardia.

23. A patient has dyspnea on exertion, tachycardia, and is pale. Lab data include hemoglobin level of 8 g/dL, hematocrit of 28%, platelet count of 80,000/mm^3, and a white blood cell count of 4500/mm^3. Which of the following is recommended for the patient?
    a. Platelets.
    b. Whole blood.
    c. Packed red blood cells.
    d. Fresh frozen plasma.

*24. Pleural effusion can be caused by increased hydrostatic pressure secondary to which one of the following conditions?
    a. Renal failure.
    b. Lymphadenopathy.
    c. Congestive heart failure.
    d. Thrombocytopenia.

* Reflects advanced oncology nursing content

*25. A patient receiving 4 mg busulfan (Myleran) for chronic myelogenous leukemia is complaining of shortness of breath, fatigue, and headache. Lab work indicates erythrocyte count, $3.3 \times 10^6/mm^3$; reticulocyte count, 0.3% of total erythrocyte count; mean corpuscular volume, 78 μm^3; hemoglobin concentration, 29 g/dL. Based on this information, the patient is diagnosed with:
  a. Microcytic hypochromic anemia.
  b. Microcytic normochromic anemia.
  c. Macrocytic normochromic anemia.
  d. Normocytic hypochromic anemia.

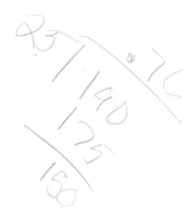

ANSWERS

1. **(b)**   A mediastinal shift will occur when the pneumothorax causes the heart and vessels to shift to the unaffected side of the pleural cavity. This will cause decreased filling of the heart, leading to decreased cardiac output.

2. **(a)**   Cool mist via an oxygen tent helps to minimize inflammation of the bronchial tissue, thus helping to prevent laryngeal edema.

3. **(c)**   Expectoration of blood is an indication of a complication of thoracentesis.

4. **(a)**   Energy conservation through pacing activities and keeping activities simple will minimize fatigue and ventilation complications, while allowing the patient some independence.

5. **(b)**   Morphine sulfate slows the respiratory rate and reduces dyspnea.

6. **(c)**   Since pneumonitis is an inflammatory response from radiation, a patient with preexisting lung inflammation would be at a higher risk for its occurrence.

7. **(a)**   Damage to the endothelial cells within the alveoli leads to inflammation and fibrosis of the alveoli.

8. **(a)**   Mild symptoms of pulmonary toxicity can be managed with cough suppressants, antipyretics, and energy conservation.

9. **(b)**   Limiting the cumulative dose of bleomycin (Blenoxane) to 400 units or less is important in preventing pulmonary fibrosis.

10. **(c)**   Capillary leak syndrome is associated with hypersensitivity reactions.

11. **(d)**   Preexisting lung disease as well as smoking history are risk factors related to the development of pulmonary fibrosis from the administration of carmustine (BCNU).

12. **(c)**   Radiation-related pulmonary toxicity generally occurs 6 to 12 weeks after the completion of treatment.

13. **(a)**   Cyanosis is a late sign of radiation-induced pulmonary toxicity.

14. **(b)**   A reduction in lung volume will be revealed by a pulmonary function test.

15. **(a)**   Albuterol is a bronchodilator that increases air flow to the lungs.

16. **(b)**   Physical signs of dyspnea are tachypnea, nostril flaring, digital clubbing.

17. **(d)**   The use of relaxation techniques can provide relief from the sensation of dyspnea.

18. **(a)**   Sudden pain may be indicative of a more serious problem.

19. **(d)**   Capillary permeability may be increased by the implantation of malignant cells on the pleural tissues, leading to inflammation and disruption of the capillary balance.

20. **(a)**   The most common malignancies that cause pleural effusion are breast, lung, and lymphoma.

21. (c)　Nitrogen mustard (Mustargen) is used as a sclerosing agent to treat pleural effusion.

22. (a)　Nonproductive cough, chest pain, and dyspnea are commonly present in patients with pleural effusion.

23. (c)　The patient is exhibiting signs and symptoms of anemia, which is treated with packed red blood cells.

*24. (c)　Congestive heart failure may cause increased hydrostatic pressure, leading to pleural effusion.

*25. (a)　The term "microcytic anemia" is used when the mean corpuscular volume is below 80 μm^3. The term "hypochromic" is used when the mean corpuscular hemoglobin concentration is less than 30 g/dL.

---

* Reflects advanced oncology nursing content

CHAPTER 16

Alterations in Circulation

QUESTIONS

1. Lymphedema of the lower extremities may result from:
    a. Radiation treatment for lung cancer.
    b. Surgical removal of the ovaries.
    c. Radiation treatment for advanced prostate cancer.
    d. Surgical removal of one kidney.

2. What is the definition of moderate arm lymphedema?
    a. A 1-cm difference in circumference from one arm to the other arm.
    b. A 2-cm difference in circumference from one arm to the other arm.
    c. A 4-cm difference in circumference from one arm to the other arm.
    d. More than 5 centimeters of difference in circumference from one arm to the other arm.

3. Which of the following statements reflects the patient's understanding of minimizing edema?
    a. "I will apply my elastic sleeve compression device in the evening for best results."
    b. "When sitting, I will rest my arms on pillows at the level of the chest."
    c. "I will institute massage therapy every day to keep my circulation in top condition."
    d. "There is no need to measure the swelling in my arm except when it is severe."

4. A common accompanying symptom of arm edema is:
    a. Redness in the affected arm.
    b. Stiffness in the unaffected limb.
    c. Numbness in the affected arm.
    d. Pain in the affected arm.

5. Which of the following chemotherapeutic agents is most associated with cardiotoxicity?
    a. Mitomycin (Mutamycin).
    b. Dactinomycin (Cosmegen).
    c. Methotrexate (MTX).
    d. Daunorubicin (Cerubidine).

6. An important nursing intervention in assessing a patient's risk for cardiotoxicity during treatment with mitoxantrone (Novantrone) is to:
    a. Assess lab values weekly.
    b. Assess for activity intolerance.
    c. Monitor electrocardiogram results weekly.
    d. Monitor the total cumulative dose the patient has received.

7. Signs and symptoms of congestive heart failure include:
    a. Nonproductive cough and dyspnea.
    b. Productive cough and neck vein distention.
    c. Productive cough and tachycardia.
    d. Nonproductive cough and splenomegaly.

8. Which of the following diagnostic procedures is recommended for assessment of chemotherapy-related cardiac toxicity?
    a. Thallium scan.
    b. Chest x-ray.
    c. Cardiac catheterization.
    d. Multigated angiogram (MUGA).

9. Symptoms of cardiac toxicity caused by paclitaxel (Taxol) include:
   a. Angina and sweating.
   b. Hypotension and bradycardia.
   c. Productive cough and hypotension.
   d. Syncope and hypotension.

10. Which of the following drugs administered concomitantly with doxorubicin (Adriamycin) may increase the cardiac effect?
    a. Cyclophosphamide (Cytoxan).
    b. Etoposide (VP-16).
    c. Cytarabine (ARA-C).
    d. Vincristine (Oncovin).

11. Which of the following classes of drugs may be used to treat cardiac symptoms caused by high-dose 5-fluorouracil (5-FU)?
    a. Diuretics.
    b. Calcium channel blockers.
    c. ACE inhibitors.
    d. Short-acting nitrates.

12. An important nursing intervention for a patient experiencing sacral edema is:
    a. Maintaining bedrest.
    b. Assessing for skin breakdown.
    c. Measuring pedal edema.
    d. Assessing skin color.

13. The primary reason albumin is administered for malignancy-related edema is to:
    a. Increase hydration status.
    b. Provide nutritional protein.
    c. Relieve electrolyte imbalance.
    d. Maintain intravascular osmotic pressure.

14. Which laboratory finding is common in a patient with malignant edema?
    a. Decreased total protein.
    b. Decreased blood urea nitrogen.
    c. Decreased creatinine clearance.
    d. Decreased potassium.

15. Discharge education for a patient with lower extremity edema should include teaching to:
    a. Alternate activity with rest periods.
    b. Increase fluid intake to 2000 mL/day.
    c. Weigh daily at the same time.
    d. Increase potassium intake.

16. Which of the following cancers is most associated with pericardial effusion?
    a. Lung cancer.
    b. Colon cancer.
    c. Melanoma.
    d. Leukemia.

17. In assessing for pericardial effusion, the nurse would expect to find which of the following clinical signs?
    a. Tachycardia and pulsus paradoxus.
    b. Bradycardia and jugular vein distention.
    c. Tachycardia and hypertension.
    d. Bradycardia and pulsus paradoxus.

18. Which diagnostic test is the most appropriate to assess for pericardial effusion?
    a. CT scan.
    b. Electrocardiogram.
    c. Chest x-ray.
    d. Echocardiogram.

19. A patient receiving mediastinal radiation for Hodgkin's disease is at risk for pericardial effusion caused by:
    a. Pericardial thickening.
    b. Decreased cardiac output.
    c. Pulmonary fibrosis.
    d. Pericardial necrosis.

20. To minimize the severity of symptoms of pericardial effusion, it is important to teach the patient to do all of the following EXCEPT:
    a. Maintain a cool environment.
    b. Elevate the head of the bed 45° to 60°.
    c. Perform relaxation exercises.
    d. Elevate lower extremities.

21. A patient with stomach cancer presents to a clinic with a platelet count of 550,000/mm^3. The nurse suspects the patient has:
    a. Autoimmune hemolytic syndrome.
    b. Polycythemia vera.
    c. Idiopathic thrombocytopenia purpura.
    d. Trousseau's syndrome.

22. Thrombophlebitis is an adverse reaction to which anticancer treatment?
    a. Mitomycin (Mutamycin).
    b. Nitrogen mustard (Mustargen).
    c. Tamoxifen (Nolvadex).
    d. Cisplatin (Platinol).

23. A patient with leukemia reports a sudden sensation of pain with paleness in his left arm. The causative factor is most likely:
    a. Arterial occlusion.
    b. Venous occlusion.
    c. Deep vein thrombosis.
    d. Subclavicular thrombosis.

*24. When a cancer patient is diagnosed with microangiopathic hemolytic anemia (MAHA), the nurse should be aware of which of the following lab values?
    a. Hemoglobin, less than 7.0 mg.
    b. Platelet count, less than 50,000.
    c. Prothrombin time, more than 16.
    d. Partial thromboplastin time, more than 34.

* Reflects advanced oncology nursing content

*25. Mrs. Miller is a patient with colon cancer who also has a history of renal disease. She takes conjugated estrogens (Premarin), cortisone (Cortone Acetate), and omeprazole (Prilosec). This patient is at an increased risk for developing:

a. Anemia.
b. Peripheral edema.
c. Arrhythmias.
d. Pleural effusion.

ANSWERS

1. **(c)**   Lymphedema in the lower extremities can be caused by advanced cancer (such as prostate cancer), which can obstruct the lymph channels. Also, radiation therapy can cause scarring, which interrupts lymph flow.

2. **(c)**   Moderate lymphedema is considered a 3- to 5-cm difference.

3. **(b)**   Elevating the affected limb to the level of the heart facilitates drainage and minimizes edema.

4. **(c)**   Numbness in the affected limb is common.

5. **(d)**   Daunorubicin (Cerubidine) can cause the heart to pump less efficiently, thus leading to cardiomyopathy.

6. **(d)**   Monitor the total cumulative dose the patient has received because a cumulative dose of 120 mg/m^2 can cause cardiac problems.

7. **(a)**   Signs and symptoms of congestive heart failure include nonproductive cough and shortness of breath.

8. **(d)**   Multigated angiogram assists in detecting ejection fraction problems, which subsequently provide information about cardiac toxicity related to chemotherapy.

9. **(b)**   Symptoms of cardiac toxicity caused by paclitaxel (Taxol) include bradycardia, hypotension, and atypical chest pain.

10. **(a)**   Cyclophosphamide (Cytoxan) can cause endothelial myocardial damage in high doses. When given with other cardiotoxic chemotherapeutic agents, the toxic effects are potentially enhanced.

11. **(b)**   Calcium channel blockers are used to treat the cardiac effects caused by high-dose 5-FU therapy.

12. **(b)**   Sacral edema can contribute to skin breakdown; thus, assessing skin integrity is an important nursing intervention.

13. **(d)**   Albumin helps to provide for intravascular osmotic pressure, which minimizes leakage of fluid into the interstitial tissues.

14. **(a)**   A decreased total protein level is common in patients with malignant edema.

15. **(c)**   It is important that patients with lower extremity edema weigh themselves at the same time daily to assess for fluid accumulation. Up to 10 pounds of fluid can accumulate before edema is noticed.

16. **(a)**   Lung cancer is most associated with pericardial effusion.

17. **(a)**   Clinical signs of pericardial effusion include tachycardia, pulsus paradoxus, peripheral edema, hypotension, and jugular vein distention.

18. **(d)**   Echocardiography provides a more accurate assessment of the extent of an effusion.

19. **(a)** Radiation to the mediastinum can cause pericardial thickening, which can contribute to an accumulation of fluid in the pericardial sac.

20. **(d)** Elevation of lower extremities does not relieve severity of symptoms related to pericardial effusion.

21. **(d)** Trousseau's syndrome is often associated with gastrointestinal cancers and causes thrombocytosis.

22. **(c)** Thrombophlebitis has been reported with tamoxifen (Nolvadex).

23. **(a)** Arterial occlusion is associated with acute, abrupt pain in the affected area with associated paleness.

*24. **(a)** A hemoglobin level of less than 7.0 mg/dL is common with microangiopathic hemolytic anemia.

*25. **(b)** Risk factors for developing edema include cardiac, renal, or liver disease as well as estrogen or steroid therapy.

* Reflects advanced oncology nursing content

ONCOLOGIC EMERGENCIES

PART V

CHAPTER 17

Metabolic Emergencies

QUESTIONS

1. Which of the following metabolic emergencies results in both thrombosis and hemorrhage?
   a. Sepsis.
   b. Tumor lysis syndrome.
   c. Disseminated intravascular coagulation (DIC).
   d. Pancytopenia.

2. Which of the following laboratory results are increased in a person with disseminated intravascular coagulation (DIC)?
   a. Fibrinogen.
   b. Platelet count.
   c. Hematocrit.
   d. Prothrombin time (PT).

3. Which of the following blood component therapies provides fibrinogen and Factor VIII, which are used in treating disseminated intravascular coagulation (DIC)?
   a. Platelets.
   b. Cryoprecipitate.
   c. Fresh frozen plasma.
   d. Immunoglobulin E.

4. The most common cause of disseminated intravascular coagulation (DIC) in persons with cancer is:
   a. Sepsis.
   b. Chemotherapy.
   c. Kidney dysfunction.
   d. Anaphylaxis.

5. To monitor potential sites for bleeding, which intervention is most appropriate?
   a. Hematest urine, stool, and emesis.
   b. Obtain weekly platelet counts.
   c. Monitor red cell morphology lab work.
   d. Weigh the client daily.

6. In the pathophysiology of septic shock, once bacteria enter the bloodstream the body reacts by releasing what cells to phagocytize bacteria?
   a. Eosinophils.
   b. Thrombocytes.
   c. Neutrophils.
   d. Interleukin-2.

7. The major side effect of antifungal therapeutic agents, such as amphotericin B, is:
   a. Leukocytosis.
   b. Rigors.
   c. Thrombocytopenia.
   d. Stomatitis.

8. Which of the following vasopressor pharmaceutical medicines is given during septic shock to increase cardiac contractility, peripheral vascular resistance, and renal blood flow?
   a. Dopamine hydrochloride (Intropin).
   b. Digoxin (Lanoxin).
   c. Norepinephrine bitartrate (Levophed).
   d. Epinephrine.

9. Hypercalcemia is defined as a serum calcium level of more than:
   a. 5 mg/dL.
   b. 8 mg/dL.
   c. 11 mg/dL.
   d. 20 mg/dL.

10. Normal levels of calcium are regulated in the body partially by the action of the gastrointestinal tract. This action occurs by means of the:
    a. Absorption of vitamin D.
    b. Production of parathyroid hormone.
    c. Excess secretion of fluids by the kidneys.
    d. Increase in prostaglandin secretion.

11. A patient has been treated for anaphylaxis. You observe an increase in weight of 7 pounds per day, a change in the urine intake and output ratio, and jugular neck vein distention. These are signs of:
    a. Respiratory distress.
    b. Anxiety.
    c. Laryngeal edema.
    d. Fluid overload.

12. At the first sign of anaphylaxis associated with chemotherapy, the nurse should:
    a. Stop the flow of the agent.
    b. Evaluate respirations.
    c. Notify the physician immediately.
    d. Lower the head of the bed.

13. To decrease respiratory distress symptoms associated with anaphylaxis, the client should be in which position?
    a. Trendelenburg.
    b. A position where the head of the bed is elevated.
    c. A position of lying flat in bed on the back.
    d. Knee-chest position.

14. The client with cancer who is at greatest risk for developing hyperkalemia is the client who has:
    a. Emphysema.
    b. Renal failure.
    c. Hypertension.
    d. Rheumatoid arthritis.

15. Which of the following medications will lower serum calcium levels?
    a. Mithramycin (Mithracin).
    b. Digoxin (Lanoxin).
    c. Cephalexin (Keflex).
    d. Pseudoephedrine (Pseudophed).

16. Neuromuscular signs and symptoms associated with hypercalcemia include:
    a. Constipation.
    b. Polydipsia.
    c. Diplopia.
    d. Hyporeflexia.

17. Prolonged hypercalcemia can result in what cardiovascular problem?
    a. Cardiac arrest.
    b. Ileus.
    c. Aortic aneurysm.
    d. Hyperlipidemia.

18. Which of the following laboratory values will be indicative of hypercalcemia?
    a. Increased serum potassium level.
    b. Increased serum sodium level.
    c. Increased serum creatinine level.
    d. Increased serum phosphorus level.

19. Which of the following nursing interventions is appropriate to maximize safety in the client with hypercalcemia who has changes in mental status?
    a. Maintain isometric exercises.
    b. Maintain bed in low position.
    c. Increased oral intake to 3000 mL per day.
    d. Assess body weight weekly.

20. The diagnostic serum test that is most beneficial in the management of syndrome of inappropriate antidiuretic hormone (SIADH) secretion is serum:
    a. Potassium.
    b. Sodium.
    c. Calcium.
    d. Bicarbonate.

21. A late sign of a syndrome of inappropriate antidiuretic hormone (SIADH) is:
    a. Headache.
    b. Vomiting.
    c. Fatigue.
    d. Seizures.

22. Seizure precautions include the client's head being:
    a. Turned to the side.
    b. Tilted back to begin CPR, if necessary.
    c. Raised to 45° in bed.
    d. Laid flat upward while lying on the back.

*23. The process of fibrinolysis in a person with disseminated intravascular coagulation (DIC) releases what products that function as anticoagulants?
    a. Platelet aggregation products.
    b. Fibrin degradation products (FDPs).
    c. Phospholipids.
    d. Antithrombin III product.

*24. A home health nurse calls you, stating that 2 days ago the patient underwent Bacillus Calmette Guerin vaccine instillation into the bladder and presents with an oral temperature of 102.4° F, heart rate of 98 beats per minute, respirations of 22 per minute, and white blood cell count of 16,000/mm^3. Based on this information, you diagnose:
    a. BCG hypersensitivity reaction.
    b. Peritonitis.
    c. Sepsis.
    d. Cardiac tamponade.

* Reflects advanced oncology nursing content

*25. Your client has an anaphylactic reaction to platinol (Cisplatin) chemotherapy. You need to give an agent that will dilate the bronchi. The agent of choice is:
a. Diphenhydramine (Benadryl).
b. Cimetidine (Tagamet).
c. Aminophylline (Theophylline).
d. Dopamine.

*26. Your client has been diagnosed with syndrome of inappropriate antidiuretic hormone (SIADH). You note that the following medication contributes to SIADH and should be discontinued:
a. Percodan.
b. Elavil.
c. Tylenol (acetaminophen).
d. Vitamin E.

ANSWERS

1. **(c)** DIC includes disruption of the endothelial membrane, resulting in coagulation and thrombosis as well as fibrinolysis, which causes clot inhibition.

2. **(d)** Prothrombin time is increased because prothrombin is the precursor to thrombin, which causes clot formation and thrombosis.

3. **(b)** Cryoprecipitate provides fibrinogen factor VIII. Fresh frozen plasma provides additional clotting factors and may aggravate DIC.

4. **(a)** Infection and sepsis are the most common causes of DIC.

5. **(a)** Hematest will monitor if blood is present or not present, thus monitoring bleeding sites.

6. **(c)** Neutrophils are the cells responsible for phagocytizing bacteria.

7. **(b)** Rigors (chills) are the major side effect of antifungal therapy.

8. **(a)** Dopamine is a vasopressor.

9. **(c)** Hypercalcemia is defined as a rise above normal levels, which are serum levels of more than 11 mg/dL.

10. **(a)** Normal levels of calcium are regulated in the GI tract by the absorption of Vitamin D.

11. **(d)** Fluid overload from anaphylaxis or its treatment is indicated by weight gain of more than 5 pounds per day, a change in the intake-output ratio, and jugular neck vein distention.

12. **(a)** Stopping the flow of the agent that is causing the anaphylaxis is the first intervention a nurse should implement.

13. **(b)** Elevation of the head of the bed decreases resistance to breathing and aids in chest expansion.

14. **(b)** Renal failure leads to a decrease in the kidneys' ability to clear calcium from the bloodstream, leading to increased serum calcium levels.

15. **(a)** Mithramycin inhibits bone resorption, thereby decreasing serum calcium levels.

16. **(d)** Hyporeflexia, weakness, confusion, personality changes, and bone pain are neuromuscular signs and symptoms of hypercalcemia.

17. **(a)** Cardiac arrest can occur as a result of high serum calcium levels.

18. **(c)** Elevated BUN and creatinine levels indicate renal failure or dysfunction; hypercalcemia and increased levels of serum potassium, sodium, and phosphorus also are indicators.

19. **(b)** Maintaining the bed in a low position with side rails up is a safety measure and placing the call light within reach is another.

20. **(b)** Serum sodium is assessed as excess production of antidiuretic hormone (ADH) from tumors results in excessive water retention and dilutional hyponatremia.

21. (d) Seizures are a late sign of SIADH, along with progressive lethargy, which can lead to coma.

22. (a) Seizure precautions include turning the client's head to the side, loosening tight clothing, promoting a safe environment, and monitoring for respiratory distress.

*23. (b) Fibrin split products (FSPs) and fibrin degradation products (FDPs) are released into the circulation during disseminated intravascular coagulation and function as anticoagulants.

*24. (c) Sepsis is a systemic inflammatory response to microorganisms and includes the parameters of fever, tachycardia, increased respiratory rate, and a white blood cell count of more than $12,000/mm^3$.

*25. (c) Aminophylline dilates bronchi, requiring the monitoring of pulse rate, rhythm, and intensity.

*26. (b) Antidepressants contribute to SIADH as do morphine and diuretics.

---

* Reflects advanced oncology nursing content

CHAPTER 18

Structural Emergencies

QUESTIONS

1. Increased intracranial pressure can be caused by:
   a. Displacement of osteoclastic activity.
   b. Obstruction of the right pulmonary bronchus.
   c. Edema of brain tissue.
   d. Decreased vascularity in the lower extremities.

2. Which of the following classifications of chemotherapeutic agents crosses the blood-brain barrier?
   a. Vinka alkaloids.
   b. Alkylating agents.
   c. Antimetabolites.
   d. Nitrosoureas.

3. The primary reason to use corticosteroids in patients with brain tumors is because corticosteroids:
   a. Decrease inflammation.
   b. Increase vascular resistance.
   c. Increase receptor activation in the true vomiting center.
   d. Induce diuresis.

4. Which of the following is an early neurologic sign of increased intracranial pressure?
   a. Coughing.
   b. Fever.
   c. Blurred vision.
   d. Widening pulse pressure.

5. Which of the following nursing interventions will help in avoiding the Valsalva maneuver?
   a. Administer narcotics around the clock.
   b. Elevate head of bed 60° to decrease venous drainage.
   c. Monitor blood pressure for widening pulse pressure.
   d. Administer stool softeners.

6. In increased intracranial pressure, what happens to the pulse pressure?
   a. It decreases or shortens.
   b. It widens or increases.
   c. The systolic pressure increases, while the diastolic pressure remains the same.
   d. It stays the same, no changes.

7. Which support service is the appropriate referral for learning to use assistive devices?
   a. Social services.
   b. Cardiac rehabilitation services.
   c. Social Security office.
   d. Physical therapy.

8. Which test is most appropriate for diagnosing and localizing spinal metastases?
   a. Magnetic resonance imaging (MRI).
   b. Myelogram without contrast.
   c. Spinal x-rays.
   d. Cerebral angiogram.

9. What is the most immediate nonpharmacologic intervention for treating spinal cord compression?
   a. Teletherapy.
   b. Brachytherapy.
   c. Surgery.
   d. Chemotherapy.

10. Clients at risk for spinal cord compression include those who have cancers that have a known affinity for metastasizing to the bone. These cancers include:
   a. Melanoma and myeloma.
   b. Cervical and ovarian.
   c. Prostate and astrocytoma.
   d. Breast and lung.

11. Which of the following structures is a thin-walled major vessel that carries venous drainage from the head and upper extremities to the heart?
   a. Aorta.
   b. Tricuspid valve.
   c. Superior vena cava.
   d. Right ventricle of the heart.

12. Obstruction of the superior vena cava causes cardiac output to:
   a. Increase.
   b. Decrease.
   c. Stay the same.
   d. Fluctuate by increasing during exercise only.

13. A client with non–small cell lung cancer comes in for his chemotherapy treatment. Your assessment indicates facial swelling on rising in the morning, redness of the conjunctivae, swelling of neck and arms, and dyspnea. These are early signs of what oncologic emergency?
   a. Spinal cord compression.
   b. Cardiac tamponade.
   c. Bronchiolitis obliterans.
   d. Superior vena cava syndrome.

14. What is the most precise test for diagnosis of cardiac tamponade?
   a. Chest x-ray.
   b. Echocardiography.
   c. Pericardiectomy.
   d. Electroencephalogram (EEG).

15. What is the main nursing diagnosis for a person with cardiac tamponade?
   a. Decreased cardiac output.
   b. Alteration in electrolyte patterns.
   c. Anxiety.
   d. Altered sexual function.

16. What is the treatment modality of choice in children and infants who have spinal cord compression?
   a. Antineoplastic therapy.
   b. Surgery.
   c. Genetic therapy.
   d. Radiation therapy.

*17. A client has a diagnosis of leukemia and presents in the emergency department with early morning headache in the frontal area. The headache is accompanied by coughing, diplopia, lethargy, and occasional vomiting. Your diagnosis indicates that this client is having what structural emergency?

    a. Syndrome of inappropriate antidiuretic hormone (SIADH).

    b. Septic shock.

    c. Increased intracranial pressure.

    d. Superior vena cava syndrome.

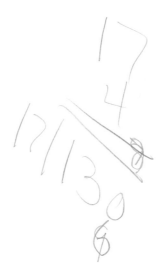

Answers

1. **(c)** Increased intracranial pressure is caused by edema of brain tissue, displacement of brain tissue by tumor, obstruction of cerebrospinal fluid, or increased angiogenesis of the brain tumor.

2. **(d)** Nitrosoureas as well as procarbazine cross the blood-brain barrier.

3. **(a)** Corticosteroids are used for their effect in decreasing inflammation and decreasing symptoms in the majority of patients with brain tumors.

4. **(c)** Neurologic signs of increased intracranial pressure include blurred vision, diplopia, visual field changes, lethargy, confusion, restlessness, and extremity drift.

5. **(d)** The Valsalva maneuver is avoided by administering stool softeners and antiemetics as well as medications to decrease headaches.

6. **(b)** Pulse pressure widens, the systolic increases and the diastolic decreases, in increased intracranial pressure.

7. **(d)** Physical therapy is the appropriate referral for learning to use assistive devices.

8. **(a)** An MRI is most appropriate for diagnosing and localizing spinal cord metastases.

9. **(a)** Teletherapy, commonly called radiation therapy, is the most immediate intervention for spinal cord compression.

10. **(d)** Spinal cord compression risk profile includes cancers that frequently metastasize to the bone. These include breast, lung, prostate, kidney, and myeloma.

11. **(c)** The superior vena cava is a vessel that carries venous drainage from the upper extremities, head, and upper thorax to the heart.

12. **(b)** Obstruction of the superior vena cava decreases cardiac output while increasing venous pressure.

13. **(d)** Signs of superior vena cava syndrome include dyspnea; hoarseness; swelling of face, neck, and arms; redness of conjunctivae; neck vein distention; and nonproductive cough.

14. **(b)** Echocardiogram shows two echos in cardiac tamponade and is the most precise diagnostic test for tamponade.

15. **(a)** Decreased cardiac output is the main diagnosis for cardiac tamponade. As pressure increases in the pericardium, left ventricular filling decreases and the ability of the heart to pump decreases, resulting in decreased cardiac output and poor systematic perfusion.

16. **(a)** Children or infants who have spinal cord compression are usually treated with antineoplastic agents, because radiation therapy can inhibit growth.

*17. **(c)** Headaches, vision problems, and gastrointestinal problems are all early signs of increased intracranial pressure (ICP), which is common in persons with brain cancer, lung or breast cancers, or leukemia.

---

* Reflects advanced oncology nursing content

SCIENTIFIC BASIS FOR PRACTICE

PART VI

CHAPTER 19

Carcinogenesis

QUESTIONS

1. An abnormal, mutated gene that converts a normal cell into a cancer cell is the definition of a(n):
   a. Tumor suppressor gene.
   b. Oncogene.
   c. Malignant cell.
   d. Promotor thymus cell (T-cell).

2. The process by which cancers arise is called:
   a. Mutation replication.
   b. Neovascularization.
   c. Initiation threshold.
   d. Carcinogenesis.

3. The formation of new blood vessels during carcinogenesis is called:
   a. Promotion.
   b. Invasion.
   c. Neovascularization.
   d. Initiation.

4. The most common route of cancer metastasis is via:
   a. Peritoneal seeding.
   b. Lymphatic spread.
   c. The blood brain barrier.
   d. Capillaries and veins.

5. What is the most common site for cancer metastasis?
   a. Brain.
   b. Bone.
   c. Heart.
   d. Lymphatics.

6. There are differences among individual cells in tumors. These differences are referred to as:
   a. Homogeneity.
   b. Heterogeneity.
   c. Modulation.
   d. Angiogenesis factors.

7. Which of the following cancers are linked to exposure to ionizing radiation?
   a. Skin cancer.
   b. Cervical cancer.
   c. Glioneuroblastomas.
   d. Colon cancer.

8. Sources of ultraviolet radiation, a carcinogen, are:
   a. Germicidal lights and coal tar.
   b. Candlelight and radiowaves.
   c. Sunlight and tanning salons.
   d. Batteries and computer microchips.

9. Which skin cancer is most commonly associated with ultraviolet radiation?
   a. Melanoma.
   b. Multiple myeloma.
   c. Ganglioneuroblastoma.
   d. Keratosis.

10. Tobacco products are chemical carcinogens. Which of the following is a tobacco product?
    a. Acetaminophen (Tylenol).
    b. Snuff.
    c. Asbestos.
    d. Benzene.

11. Diethylstilbestrol is a drug that is a known carcinogen for what type of cancer?
    a. Ovarian.
    b. Prostate.
    c. Lung.
    d. Vaginal.

12. Invasion of the bone marrow by cancer cells compromises the immune system by decreasing the production of:
    a. Thrombocytes.
    b. Red blood cells.
    c. Ionized calcium.
    d. Lymphocytes.

13. Which of the following classifications of chemotherapy agents can increase the incidence of malignancy?
    a. Alkylating agents.
    b. Nitrosoureas.
    c. Antifungal agents.
    d. Hormones.

14. The hepatitis B virus (HBV) is strongly associated with what type of cancer?
    a. Adult T-cell leukemia.
    b. Hepatocellular carcinoma.
    c. Squamous cell carcinoma.
    d. Adenocarcinoma of the colon.

15. The human papillomavirus (HPV) is strongly associated with which type of cancer?
    a. T-cell lymphoma.
    b. Burkitt's lymphoma.
    c. Cervical cancer.
    d. Prostate cancer.

16. A tumor of the eye to which a person may have a genetic predisposition is called:
    a. Wilms' tumor.
    b. Fanconi's anemia.
    c. Neurofibromatosis.
    d. Retinoblastoma.

17. The term that describes an unusual number of chromosomes present in a cancer cell is:
    a. Polymorphism.
    b. Aneuploidy.
    c. Pleomorphism.
    d. Hyperchromatism.

18. Which oncofetal antigen level is usually elevated in colorectal cancers?
    a. Carcinoembryonic antigen (CEA).
    b. Alpha-fetoprotein (AFP).
    c. Human chorionic gonadotropin (hCG).
    d. Beta-2 antigen (B-2A).

19. Which of the following cells has a high mitotic index?
    a. Cervical cells.
    b. Bone marrow cells.
    c. Dermatomes.
    d. Hepatic cells.

20. Which of the following grades of tumors is the best indicator of cells that are well differentiated and low grade?
    a. Grade I.
    b. Grade II.
    c. Grade III.
    d. Grade IV.

21. The average doubling time of most primary tumors is?
    a. Less than 3 weeks.
    b. 2 to 3 months.
    c. 6 months.
    d. 1 to 2 years.

22. The centers of tumors are often necrotic. The necrosis is caused by:
    a. Loss of protein.
    b. Loss of epithelial tissue support.
    c. Vitamin deficiencies.
    d. Absence of vascularity.

23. The term used to describe cells that have abnormal cytologic features that are often associated with premalignant change is:
    a. Atrophy.
    b. Hyperplasia.
    c. Dysplasia.
    d. Hypertrophy.

24. The removal of tissue or fluid without general anesthesia includes what type of biopsy?
    a. Incisional.
    b. Excisional.
    c. Halsted cytology.
    d. Lumpectomy.

*25. Your client is about to have adjuvant radiation therapy to his left leg sarcoma before the primary treatment of chemotherapy is begun. The appropriate term for the radiation to be given is:
    a. Primary treatment.
    b. Additional therapy.
    c. Neoadjuvant treatment.
    d. Prophylactic treatment.

---

* Reflects advanced oncology nursing content

*26. You are hired to educate female workers at an occupational site about avoidance of known carcinogens and on self-examination for early cancer detection. Which of the following topics should you include?
   a. Asbestos and sun exposure, breast and vulvar self-exam.
   b. Gasoline exposure and testes self-exam.
   c. Tobacco exposure and colon self-exam.
   d. Candy wrapper exposure and cervical self-exam.

*27. You are about to teach a client about his treatment of intravenous combination chemo-therapy, which includes vincristine, cisplatin, and methotrexate. Your teaching will discuss those cells that are less sensitive to the effects of chemotherapy because of their low mitotic rate. The cells include:
   a. Brain and epithelial cells.
   b. Bone and neural tissue cells.
   c. Hepatic and squamous cells.
   d. Hair follicle and gastrointestinal tract cells.

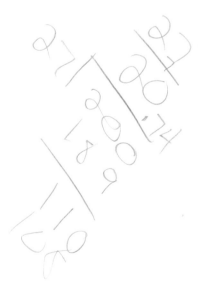

ANSWERS

1. **(b)** An oncogene is an abnormal gene that converts a normal cell into a cancer cell. Examples include the p53 tumor suppressor gene commonly found in colorectal, breast, and lung cancers and the *ras* oncogene found in pancreatic, colorectal, and thyroid cancers.

2. **(d)** Carcinogenesis is the process by which cancers arise and usually involves a series of steps that differ for each type of cancer.

3. **(c)** Neovascularization is defined as the formation of new blood vessels.

4. **(d)** Metastasis most commonly occurs via blood capillaries or veins, although it may also occur via the lymphatics and through seeding, as in the peritoneal cavity.

5. **(b)** The bones are the most common site for cancer metastasis.

6. **(b)** Heterogeneity is the term that applies to differences among cancer cells in a tumor. Heterogeneity increases as tumor growth increases.

7. **(a)** Ionized radiation exposure is linked to skin cancer, thyroid cancer, leukemia, lung cancer, breast cancer, and osteosarcomas.

8. **(c)** Sources of ultraviolet radiation include sunlight, tanning salons, and industrial welding arcs and germicidal lights.

9. **(a)** Melanoma, basal cell, and squamous cell are the most common types of skin cancer caused by ultraviolet radiation.

10. **(b)** Snuff, chewing tobacco, and cigarette, pipe, and cigar smoke are all tobacco products.

11. **(d)** Vaginal cancer is linked to diethylstilbestrol.

12. **(d)** Invasion of the bone marrow by cancer cells decreases the production of lymphocytes, thereby compromising the immune system.

13. **(a)** Alkylating agents are known to increase the incidence of cancer, in particular leukemia and lymphoma.

14. **(b)** Hepatitis B virus (HBV) is associated with hepatocellular carcinoma.

15. **(c)** Human papillomavirus (HPV) is associated with cervical and genital cancer.

16. **(d)** Retinoblastoma is a cancer of the eye that has a genetic predisposition. It usually occurs in infants and children.

17. **(b)** Aneuploidy is defined as an unusual number of chromosomes.

18. **(a)** CEA is most often expressed in colorectal, breast, and lung cancers.

19. **(b)** Bone marrow cells, GI cells, and hair follicle cells all have a high mitotic index.

20. **(a)** Grade I cells are well differentiated and are known as low-grade cells.

21. **(b)** The average doubling time of primary tumors is about 8 to 12 weeks, or 2 to 3 months.

22. **(d)**   Necrosis in tissue is caused by loss of blood supply, i.e., absence of vascularity.

23. **(c)**   Dysplasia is a part of the cellular growth process that describes cytologic features with premalignant changes.

24. **(a)**   Incisional biopsies include aspiration, fine-needle, and punch biopsies, in which general anesthesia is NOT used.

*25. **(c)**   Neoadjuvant treatment is a term used to signify adjuvant therapy given before the primary treatment.

*26. **(a)**   Occupational carcinogens include asbestos, chemicals, sun, and tobacco. Self-exam for females includes breast, skin, oral cavity, and vulvar area.

*27. **(b)**   Bone and neural tissue all have a very low mitotic rate and, therefore, are less sensitive to the effects of chemotherapeutic agents.

---

* Reflects advanced oncology nursing content

20

Immunology

QUESTIONS

1. The development of blood cells, known as hematopoiesis, begins with a single cell. This single cell is called a:
   a. Thymus-induced B-cell.
   b. Cytokine protein messenger.
   c. Pluripotent stem cell.
   d. Lymphocyte.

2. What type of stem cells mature into red blood cells and platelets?
   a. T-cells (thymus).
   b. B-cells (bursa).
   c. Lymphoid.
   d. Myeloid.

3. The majority of white blood cells are what type of granulocyte?
   a. Neutrophils.
   b. Basophils.
   c. Eosinophils.
   d. Monocytes.

4. Neutrophils and macrophages destroy bacteria, viruses, and pathogens that enter the body. This process of destruction is known as:
   a. Natural killer cell response.
   b. Monocytic survey.
   c. Phagocytosis.
   d. Inflammatory response.

5. Tissue-specific macrophages found in the liver are called:
   a. Synovial cells.
   b. Kupffer cells.
   c. Histiocytes.
   d. Bradykinins.

6. Antigen-antibody reaction in the body is a result of what type of immunity?
   a. T-cell or cell-mediated immunity.
   b. B-cell or bursa-cell immunity.
   c. Opsonization immunity.
   d. Complement immunity.

7. What is the term used to describe proteins that are secreted to communicate messages to other cells?
   a. Natural killer cells.
   b. Antigens.
   c. Cytokines.
   d. Complement proteins.

8. Which of the following best describes a person with a failed immune system?
   a. Elderly, malnourished, undergoing chemotherapy.
   b. Stressed adolescent who eats hamburgers for every meal.
   c. 32-year-old with rheumatoid arthritis.
   d. 60-year-old male postprostatectomy.

*9. In the cellular exudate stage of inflammation, or stage II, loss of function, such as that of a toe, may occur. This loss of function is primarily caused by:
   a. More fluid moving to the inflamed area.
   b. Increased production of monocytes by the bone marrow.
   c. Stimulation of tumor necrosis factor (TNF).
   d. Histamine release.

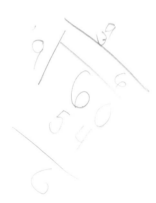

ANSWERS

1. **(c)** Pluripotent stem cell is a single cell that begins the development of blood cells, or hematopoiesis.

2. **(d)** Stem cells are committed to become either myeloid stem cells that mature into RBCs and platelets or lymphoid stem cells that mature into six types of WBCs.

3. **(a)** Neutrophils represent 62% of all white blood cells, which makes them the most numerous of granulocytes.

4. **(c)** Phagocytosis is the process whereby neutrophils and macrophages destroy bacteria, viruses, and other foreign pathogens or materials.

5. **(b)** Kupffer cells are specific tissue macrophages that are found in the liver and destroy invading pathogens.

6. **(a)** T-cell or cell-mediated immunity is responsible for antigen-antibody reactions, creating memory cells for future antigen exposure.

7. **(c)** Cytokine is the term used to describe proteins that are secreted to communicate messages to other cells.

8. **(a)** Elderly, malnourished, chronically ill, immunocompromised, and stressed individuals are at the greatest risk for a failed immune system.

*9. **(a)** During stage II of the inflammation process, cellular exudate develops with a corresponding increase of fluid into the area, causing swelling and loss of function of body parts, such as a toe.

* Reflects advanced oncology nursing content

21

Genetics

QUESTIONS

1. How many chromosomes make up the human body?
   a. 10.
   b. 22.
   c. 30.
   d. 46.

2. The process of making RNA from DNA is called:
   a. Translation.
   b. Transcription.
   c. Transportation.
   d. Translocation.

3. Which type of genes are necessary for normal cellular growth and regulation?
   a. Apoptosis genes.
   b. Telomerase genes.
   c. Tumor necrosis genes.
   d. Proto-oncogenes.

4. When susceptibility to cancer is the result of one altered gene from each parent, the genetic inheritance is termed:
   a. Autosomal recessive.
   b. Autosomal dominant.
   c. A nonsense mutation.
   d. A polymorphic mutation.

5. A genetic testing laboratory in the United States should have a laboratory director who is certified by the:
   a. Association of Genetic Researchers.
   b. Alliance of Geneticists and Sequencers.
   c. American Board of Medical Genetics.
   d. Association of Physician Directors and Managers.

6. Which of the following is part of the universal criteria for genetic testing?
   a. No family history required.
   b. No need to have a test that can be interpreted.
   c. Informed consent required.
   d. Every client is appropriate for genetic testing.

7. BRCA-1 and BRCA-2 are genes associated with what type of cancer?
   a. Lung.
   b. Breast.
   c. Thyroid.
   d. Leukemia.

8. What type of gene therapy includes the introduction of a functioning gene into the egg or sperm so the transmission of the genetic alteration does not occur?
   a. Germline gene therapy.
   b. Somatic gene therapy.
   c. Translational gene therapy.
   d. Chromatid gene therapy.

9. What is the name of the psychological guilt experienced by clients who have not inherited the genetic cancer alteration that is present in other close family members?
    a. Transmitter guilt.
    b. Heightened guilt.
    c. Guilt of regret and anger.
    d. Survivor guilt.

10. The development of a family tree in genetic assessment is called a:
    a. Pedigree.
    b. Genetic hierarchy.
    c. Risks and benefits tree.
    d. Discrimination chart.

11. Confirmation of family history for cancers is determined by:
    a. The client's verbal response.
    b. Newspaper obituaries.
    c. Death certificates.
    d. Pathology records.

*12. You are about to assess a client's genetic pedigree. Which of the following is a complete component of a pedigree?
    a. Two-generation family history.
    b. Age at death.
    c. Primary site of cancer(s).
    d. Number of live children.

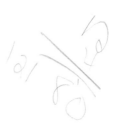

ANSWERS

1. **(d)**   46 chromosomes, 23 pairs, make up the human body.

2. **(b)**   Transcription is the process of making RNA from DNA; translation is the process of making proteins from RNA.

3. **(d)**   Proto-oncogenes are necessary for normal cell growth and regulation. Alteration in proto-oncogenes leads to uncontrolled cell growth.

4. **(a)**   Autosomal recessive inheritance is a result of one altered gene from *each* parent. Autosomal dominant inheritance is a result of one altered gene from *either* parent.

5. **(c)**   Genetic testing laboratories should meet the criteria of the Clinical Laboratory Improvement Act (CLIA) and have a Director certified by the American Board of Medical Genetics.

6. **(c)**   The universal criteria for genetic testing includes informed consent, family history, test performed that can be interpreted, and the fact that not every client is appropriate for genetic testing of inherited cancers.

7. **(b)**   BRCA-1 and BRCA-2 are autosomal dominant genes inherited in breast cancer, ovarian cancer, prostate cancer, colon cancer, and pancreatic cancer.

8. **(a)**   Germline gene therapy introduces functioning genes into the egg or sperm to prevent genetic transmission. Somatic gene therapy introduces a functioning gene into a somatic cell to replace a certain dysfunctional gene.

9. **(d)**   Survivor guilt is the term used to describe the psychological impact on a client who has been genetically tested for cancer but who is found not to carry the gene that a close family member carries.

10. **(a)**   Pedigree is the term used to refer to the development of a family tree in genetic assessment.

11. **(d)**   Pathology records are used to confirm family history of cancer because they are highly reliable.

*12. **(c)**   Assessment of genetic pedigree includes a three-generation history, primary site, age at diagnosis, previous surgery to reduce risk, pregnancy loss, birth defects, race, ethnicity, health problems, and environmental and occupational exposures.

---

* Reflects advanced oncology nursing content

22

Nursing Care of the Client with Breast Cancer

QUESTIONS

1. Which of the following is the most common invasive type of breast cancer?
   a. Ductal carcinoma.
   b. Lobular carcinoma in situ.
   c. Inflammatory breast cancer.
   d. Paget's disease.

2. Which of the following hormone receptor assays are routinely implemented on breast tumor specimens?
   a. Aneuploid receptor.
   b. S-phase receptor.
   c. Estrogen receptor.
   d. p53 gene receptor.

3. The Mammography Quality Standards Act is a federal law that requires:
   a. Mammography facilities to be certified.
   b. Everyone over the age of 50 to have a mammogram.
   c. Free mammograms for persons over the age of 75 years.
   d. Ultrasound imaging to be done on all suspected positive mammograms.

4. A stereotactic fine-needle aspiration is used in what type of breast cancer?
   a. Nonpalpable lesion.
   b. Palpable lesion of more than 5 cm.
   c. Excisional biopsy lesion.
   d. Incisional biopsy lesion.

5. Which of the following is a breast-conserving surgical procedure for breast cancer?
   a. Modified mastectomy.
   b. Subcutaneous mastectomy.
   c. Total mastectomy.
   d. Lumpectomy.

6. Long-term effects on the lung after radiation therapy for breast cancer include:
   a. Cardiac tamponade.
   b. Pneumonitis.
   c. Pulmonary emboli.
   d. Paralytic ileus.

7. Which of the following women with breast cancer should have the highest response rate to hormonal therapy?
   a. ER (estrogen receptor) positive only.
   b. PR (progesterone receptor) positive only.
   c. ER and PR negative.
   d. ER and PR positive.

8. The name of the surgical procedure that achieves ovarian ablation is called:
   a. Hysterectomy.
   b. Oophorectomy.
   c. Cervical conization.
   d. Vulvectomy.

9. Which stage of breast cancer will most likely require local treatment for palliation?
   a. Stage I.
   b. Stage II.
   c. Stage III.
   d. Stage IV.

10. Which of the following statements is TRUE regarding family history of breast cancer?
    a. Risk is increased if first-degree relative developed breast cancer before menopause.
    b. Over 50% of breast cancers are caused by genetic factors.
    c. Mutation on chromosome number 26 conveys increased risk.
    d. Risk increases threefold to fourfold for females if a male in the family has had breast cancer.

11. Secondary risk factors for breast cancer include exposure to excessive ionizing radiation, such as from:
    a. Usual dental x-rays.
    b. Computer work.
    c. Multiple fluoroscopies.
    d. Microwave ovens.

12. The majority of breast lumps are:
    a. Painless.
    b. Painful.
    c. Malignant.
    d. Discovered by health care providers.

13. What is the most common diagnostic test used to determine bone metastasis in a person with breast cancer?
    a. Bone scan.
    b. Magnetic resonance imaging (MRI).
    c. Angiogram.
    d. Doppler ultrasound.

14. To prevent fluid accumulation under the chest wall incision after mastectomy, surgical drains are utilized. When should the drains be discontinued?
    a. After 48 hours.
    b. After 24 hours.
    c. When output is less than 120 mL/24 hours.
    d. When output is less than 30 mL/24 hours.

15. A nurse should educate a client that altered arm and breast sensations, such as numbness of the arm and phantom breast sensation, after mastectomy may last for:
    a. Days.
    b. Weeks.
    c. Months.
    d. Years.

16. Which of the following is an effective post-axillary dissection exercise for women after mastectomy?
    a. Hand wall climbing.
    b. Needlepoint sewing.
    c. Calf rodeo roping.
    d. 2-pound bench press.

*17. Which of the following are the worst prognostic factors for a woman with breast cancer?
     a. ER positive hormone receptors, 2-cm tumor, well differentiated.
     b. High S-phase, 3-cm tumor, six positive lymph nodes.
     c. Low grade, well differentiated, 12 positive lymph nodes.
     d. 4-cm tumor, poorly differentiated, 10 positive lymph nodes.

*18. You have a patient with recurrent stage III ductal breast carcinoma who has failed treatment on anthracyclines and now has a pathologic fracture of the right humerus. The next course of chemotherapy offered should include:
     a. Cyclophosphamide (Cytoxan).
     b. Tamoxifen (Nolvadex).
     c. Interleukin-2 (IL-2).
     d. Taxoids.

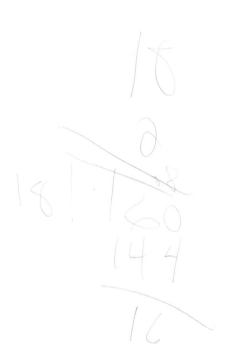

ANSWERS

1. **(a)**   Ductal carcinoma accounts for 70% of all breast cancers, and it is an invasive type.

2. **(c)**   Estrogen and progesterone receptor assays are common hormone receptor assays done on breast tumor specimens.

3. **(a)**   The Mammography Quality Standards Act is a federal law that requires all facilities that do mammograms to be certified.

4. **(a)**   Stereotactic fine-needle aspiration is used on nonpalpable breast lesions because it can locate the nonpalpable abnormality by using specially designed computer mammography equipment.

5. **(d)**   Lumpectomy and segmental resections, also called partial mastectomy, are breast-conserving surgeries.

6. **(b)**   Pneumonitis, rib fractures, hyperpigmentation of the skin, soft-tissue fibrosis, and brachial plexopathy are possible long-term effects from radiation therapy for breast cancer.

7. **(d)**   Women with breast cancer who are both ER and PR positive have a more than 70% positive response to hormonal therapy.

8. **(b)**   Oophorectomy is the term for surgical ovarian ablation.

9. **(d)**   Stage IV breast cancer requires treatment with systemic chemotherapy or hormone therapy AND local treatment(s) for palliation.

10. **(a)**   Risk factors for breast cancer include female gender, over age 75 years, personal history, first-degree relative who had breast cancer (especially if premenopausal at diagnosis), and presence of BRCA-1 and BRCA-2 gene mutation.

11. **(c)**   Exposure to excessive ionizing radiation from multiple fluoroscopies, radiation to the head and neck or chest for mastitis or acne, and radiation therapy for treatment of Hodgkin's disease are secondary risk factors in the development of breast cancer.

12. **(a)**   Most breast lumps are painless and only 25% are malignant.

13. **(a)**   A bone scan is the most common diagnostic test used to assess for bone metastasis from breast cancer.

14. **(d)**   Surgical drains, after mastectomy, are removed after 1 week or when drainage is less than 30 mL/day.

15. **(d)**   Altered sensations may last for years after mastectomy. These include arm numbness and tingling, chest wall void of feeling, and phantom breast sensation.

16. **(a)**   Effective post-axillary dissection exercises after mastectomy include arm swings, hand wall climbing, pulley exercises, and circular turning of rope tied to a door handle.

*17. **(d)** Poor prognostic factors for women with breast cancer include large tumor size; high grade; poorly differentiated; increased number of positive lymph nodes; ER/PR negative; inflammatory breast cancer; aneuploid; and high S-phase.

*18. **(d)** Taxoids such as paclitaxel (Taxol) and docetaxel (Taxotere) are used for anthracycline-resistant metastatic breast cancer.

* Reflects advanced oncology nursing content

23

Nursing Care
of the Client
with Urinary Cancer

QUESTIONS

1. The most common risk factor for kidney cancer is:
    a.   Increased dietary protein.
    b.   High serum estrogen.
    c.   Cigarette smoking.
    d.   Previous exposure to ultraviolet radiation.

2. Which one of the following cancers is radioresistant?
    a.   Colon cancer.
    b.   Hodgkin's disease.
    c.   Bone metastasis from breast cancer.
    d.   Kidney cancer.

3. What physical examination sign would indicate possible renal cancer?
    a.   Hematuria.
    b.   Chest pain.
    c.   Diarrhea.
    d.   Chronic cough.

4. What is the most common surgical procedure to treat cancer of the kidney?
    a.   Ureterostomy.
    b.   Nephrectomy.
    c.   Hepatic ligation.
    d.   Oophorectomy.

5. Your client is 48 hours postnephrectomy from newly diagnosed kidney cancer. The client awakens at 2 AM complaining of abdominal distention and you auscultate no bowel sounds. Your assessment indicates:
    a.   Hemorrhage.
    b.   Constipation.
    c.   Acute surgical pain.
    d.   Paralytic ileus.

6. Which of the following is an intravesical chemotherapy used to treat bladder cancer?
    a.   Thiotepa.
    b.   Cyclophosphamide (Cytoxan).
    c.   Methotrexate (Mexate).
    d.   Medroxyprogesterone acetate (Depo-Provera).

7. Which of the following is a urinary diversion?
    a.   Ileostomy.
    b.   Colostomy.
    c.   Ileal conduit.
    d.   Proctostomy.

8. A urinary diversion should produce urine:
    a.   Right after surgery.
    b.   Within 12 hours after surgery.
    c.   Within 24 hours after surgery.
    d.   Within 48 hours after surgery.

9. A stoma that is purple in color indicates:
   a. A normal stoma.
   b. Necrosis.
   c. Hemorrhage.
   d. Impaired circulation.

10. What food should a urinary diversion client avoid to prevent malodorous urine?
    a. Chocolate chip cookies.
    b. Peanut butter.
    c. Asparagus.
    d. Jelly beans.

11. You should educate persons with a urinary diversion to take what vitamin in order to avoid malodorous urine?
    a. Vitamin A.
    b. Vitamin B_6.
    c. Vitamin C.
    d. Vitamin E.

12. An ileal conduit pouch should be changed on a regular basis to avoid peristomal skin breakdown. A regular basis means:
    a. Daily.
    b. Every 2 to 3 days.
    c. Every 3 to 7 days.
    d. Every other week.

13. The highest rate of prostate cancer in males in the world is among:
    a. Caucasians.
    b. Asians.
    c. Hispanics.
    d. African-Americans.

14. The most effective method of detecting prostate cancer early is by doing a:
    a. Digital rectal examination (DRE).
    b. Serum prostate antibody test.
    c. Flat plate x-ray of the abdomen.
    d. Lymphangiogram.

15. Elevated serum alkaline phosphate levels in a male with prostate cancer indicate:
    a. Urinary metastasis.
    b. Lung metastasis.
    c. Bone metastasis.
    d. Colon metastasis.

16. The major complication associated with surgical treatment for prostate cancer is:
    a. Impotence.
    b. Hemorrhage.
    c. Urinary incontinence.
    d. Priapism.

17. To alleviate cystitis associated with radiation therapy for prostate cancer, the nurse should educate the client to:
    a. Ambulate at least three times per day.
    b. Avoid carrying objects over 2 pounds in weight.
    c. Drink at least 2 liters of fluids daily.
    d. Avoid drinking milk and eating yogurt.

18. Radiation therapy for the treatment of prostate cancer can cause proctitis. The symptoms of proctitis are:
    a. Cramps, diarrhea, rectal pain.
    b. Constipation and rectal itching.
    c. Loss of rectal sphincter tone and hypercalcemia.
    d. Urinary incontinence and abdominal pain.

19. Testicular implants are a suggested alternative after what surgical procedure?
    a. Oophorectomy.
    b. Orchiectomy.
    c. Transurethral radical prostatectomy.
    d. Abdominal peritoneal resection.

20. A client with proctitis should *avoid* what type of diet?
    a. High-protein.
    b. Low-fat, low-residue.
    c. Full liquid.
    d. High-residue.

21. To continue to monitor the progress of prostate cancer, after prostatectomy, which of the following lab values is assessed?
    a. Human chorionic gonadotropin (HCG), plasma.
    b. Serum glucose.
    c. Carcinogenic embryonic antigen (CEA).
    d. Serum prostate-specific antigen (PSA).

22. What emergency treatment is used for spinal cord compression caused by metastasis from prostate cancer?
    a. Single-dose chemotherapy.
    b. Combination chemotherapy.
    c. Radiation therapy.
    d. Interleukin-3 therapy.

23. Luteinizing hormone–releasing hormones, such as leuprolide or goserelin, are used as treatment for prostate cancer because they:
    a. Increase estrogen production.
    b. Increase progesterone production.
    c. Decrease human chorionic gonadotropin hormone.
    d. Decrease testosterone production.

24. Complications from radiation therapy for prostate cancer include:
    a. Proctitis and paralytic ileus.
    b. Acute cystitis and impotence.
    c. Constipation and priapism.
    d. Anemia and colitis.

*25. You are doing a workup on a 66-year-old male who may have prostate cancer. What is the correct order of the workup?
- a. Serum acid phosphatase, serum PSA, digital rectal exam.
- b. Digital rectal exam, serum PSA, serum acid phosphatase.
- c. Serum alkaline phosphatase, digital rectal exam, serum acid phosphatase.
- d. CT scan lymph nodes, digital rectal exam, serum acid phosphatase.

*26. Your client is 36 hours postcystectomy with an ileal conduit. Normal saline is being given intravenously at 150 mL/hr, diet is full liquid, and fever is 101.8° F. You note an area of drainage at the abdominal wound site and abdominal tenderness upon light palpation. Urinary output has decreased from 140 mL/hr to 50 mL/hr. You suspect:
- a. Peritonitis.
- b. Capillary leak syndrome.
- c. Paralytic ileus.
- d. Renal failure.

*27. You meet a new client who is a 55-year-old Egyptian male, works as a painter, has smoked two packs of cigarettes a day for 40 years, uses artificial sweetener in three cups of coffee per day, and complains of gross but painless hematuria. The client probably has what type of cancer?
- a. Renal cell.
- b. Lung.
- c. Bladder.
- d. Colon.

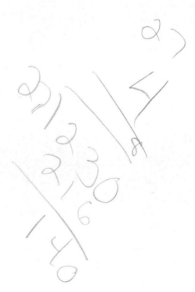

ANSWERS

1. **(c)**   Cigarette smoking is the most common risk factor for kidney cancer. Other risk factors include phenacetin intake, coal tars, asbestos, and printing ink made with lead pigments.

2. **(d)**   Kidney cancer is radioresistant.

3. **(a)**   Hematuria is a late sign of renal cancer in about half of all cases. Other signs include dull abdominal ache, abdominal mass, fever, weight loss, elevated cardiac QRS wave, and anemia.

4. **(b)**   Nephrectomy is a common surgical procedure to treat kidney cancer.

5. **(d)**   Paralytic ileus is a common occurrence after nephrectomy that results from intestinal manipulation during surgery. The signs include abdominal distention and lack of bowel sounds.

6. **(a)**   Common intravesical chemotherapy used to treat bladder cancer includes thiotepa, doxorubicin, BCG, or mitomycin-C.

7. **(c)**   An ileal conduit is a urinary diversion required to treat some stages of bladder cancer.

8. **(a)**   A urinary diversion, unlike a fecal diversion, should produce urine right after surgery.

9. **(d)**   A purple-colored stoma indicates impaired circulation, whereas black coloration indicates necrosis. Both require immediate attention.

10. **(c)**   Asparagus, fish, and carbonated beverages cause malodorous urine in persons with urinary diversions.

11. **(c)**   Vitamin C intake will decrease odor in urinary diversion output.

12. **(c)**   An ileal conduit pouch is changed every 3 to 7 days to avoid peristomal skin breakdown.

13. **(d)**   African-Americans have the highest incidence of prostate cancer in the world; Asians are at low risk.

14. **(a)**   Digital rectal examination is the most effective method for detecting prostate cancer.

15. **(c)**   Increased serum levels of alkaline phosphatase indicate bone metastasis in a client with prostate cancer.

16. **(a)**   Impotence is the major side effect associated with surgical treatment for prostate cancer. Other side effects include urinary incontinence and stricture formation in the urethra.

17. **(c)**   To alleviate cystitis associated with radiation for prostate cancer, have the client drink at least 2 liters of fluid per day.

18. **(a)**   Symptoms of proctitis include cramps, diarrhea, and rectal pain.

19. **(b)**   Testicular implants are often suggested after surgical removal of the testes (orchiectomy) for persons treated for cancer.

20. **(d)**   A person with proctitis should avoid a high-residue diet and should take antidiarrhea medications as prescribed.

21. **(d)** Prostate cancer is monitored by assessing periodic serum levels of prostate-specific antigen (PSA).

22. **(c)** Radiation therapy is the treatment of choice for spinal cord compression in adults.

23. **(d)** Luteinizing hormone–releasing hormones are used to treat prostate cancer because they decrease testosterone production.

24. **(b)** Complications associated with radiation therapy for prostate cancer include acute cystitis, impotence, and proctitis.

*25. **(a)** A correct workup for prostate cancer includes drawing serum levels first, followed by the digital rectal exam, because trauma to the prostate causes release of acid phosphatase into the bloodstream.

*26. **(a)** Peritonitis can be associated with anastomotic leak and includes the signs of abdominal tenderness or distention, fever, sudden decrease in urinary output, or abdominal wound drainage.

*27. **(c)** Bladder cancer risk includes male gender; over 75 years old; African or Egyptian origin; exposure to dyes, paint, rubber, or leather; smoking history; use of artificial sweetener; gross painless hematuria; and burning or urgency.

* Reflects advanced oncology nursing content

CHAPTER 24

Nursing Care of the Client with Lung Cancer

QUESTIONS

1. Which of the following is a TRUE statement about the incidence of lung cancer?
   a. The incidence is increasing in men.
   b. The incidence is decreasing in women.
   c. Lung cancer is the leading type of cancer for both men and women in the U.S.
   d. The incidence rate for lung cancer has remained the same for the last 50 years.

2. An increase in lung cancer deaths in women is attributed to an increase in:
   a. Radon exposure.
   b. Smoking cigarettes.
   c. Obesity.
   d. Sun exposure.

3. Which of the following pulmonary tests are done to localize and perform a biopsy on a lesion in the lung?
   a. Thoracentesis.
   b. Computed tomography (CT) scan.
   c. Mediastinoscopy.
   d. Bronchoscopy.

4. The current treatment of choice for small cell lung cancer is:
   a. Radiation alone.
   b. Combination chemotherapy.
   c. Alpha-interferon alone.
   d. Surgical resection and interleukin-3.

5. The treatment of choice for non–small cell cancer of the lung is:
   a. Surgery.
   b. Brachytherapy.
   c. Single-dose chemotherapy with cyclophosphamide (Cytoxan).
   d. Beta-interferon.

6. For which of the following cancers is there no known reliable screening method?
   a. Prostate.
   b. Breast.
   c. Colon.
   d. Lung.

7. Which of the following is a pulmonary sign or symptom that might be seen in clients who have lung cancer?
   a. Cough.
   b. Shoulder pain.
   c. Vomiting.
   d. Fever.

8. Your patient has chest tubes in the left lung for 18 hours following a resection for lung cancer. On making rounds, you note an absence of fluctuations in the water seal chamber and a lack of fluid drainage in the collection chamber. These signs indicate a(n):
   a. Obstruction.
   b. Air leak.
   c. Positive occlusive seal at the insertion site.
   d. Accumulation of some debris in the collection chamber.

9. Your client is to have a left pneumonectomy tomorrow to treat lung cancer. Your teaching should include that after surgery the client may NOT lie in what position?
    a. Flat on the back.
    b. On the left side.
    c. On the right side.
    d. There are no restrictions on how to lie.

10. Lung cancer can metastasize to the brain, bone, or liver. What signs or symptoms would indicate possible liver metastasis?
    a. Bone pain.
    b. Changes in personality.
    c. Kussmaul breathing pattern.
    d. Jaundice.

*11. Twelve hours after surgery, your client, who has chest tubes, begins having shortness of breath. Your assessment indicates absent breath sounds unilaterally and tracheal deviation. Your assessment indicates the client has a(n):
    a. Pulmonary emboli.
    b. Abdominal aortic aneurysm.
    c. Respiratory arrest.
    d. Pneumothorax.

ANSWERS

1. **(c)**   Lung cancer is the leading cause of cancer for both men and women in the United States.

2. **(b)**   The increase in deaths of women from lung cancer is attributed to increased cigarette smoking.

3. **(d)**   A bronchoscopy is done to localize and perform a biopsy on a lung lesion.

4. **(b)**   Small cell lung cancer is treated with combination chemotherapy with or without prophylactic cranial radiation.

5. **(a)**   Lobectomy or pneumonectomy are surgical treatments of choice for non–small cell lung cancer.

6. **(d)**   Cancers of the lung and kidney have no known reliable screening methods.

7. **(a)**   Cough, dyspnea, hemoptysis, and pneumonia are pulmonary signs and symptoms of lung cancer.

8. **(a)**   Chest tube obstruction is diagnosed by absence of fluctuations in the water seal chamber and a lack of fluid drainage in the collection chambers.

9. **(c)**   After pneumonectomy, a client should lie either flat or on the operative side to protect remaining lung tissue.

10. **(d)**   Jaundice is a sign of liver metastasis.

*11. **(d)**   Signs of a pneumothorax include absent breath sounds unilaterally, increased shortness of breath, and tracheal deviation.

* Reflects advanced oncology nursing content

Nursing Care of the Client with Cancer of the Gastrointestinal Tract

QUESTIONS

1. Which of the following statements is TRUE regarding esophageal cancer?
    a. Routine screening is done worldwide.
    b. The only type of esophageal cancer is adenocarcinoma.
    c. Disease is often systemic at diagnosis.
    d. Lymph node involvement is extremely rare, less than 1% of cases.

2. Preoperative pulmonary function values for surgical procedures in esophageal cancer recommend that a client's forced expiratory volume (FEV) be at least:
    a. 20%.
    b. 32%.
    c. 50%.
    d. 70%.

3. The typical treatment for esophageal cancer in most current trials includes:
    a. Combination chemotherapy with radiation therapy.
    b. Surgery only.
    c. Teletherapy with alpha-interferon.
    d. Single-drug chemotherapy with cesium implants.

4. Prognosis for esophageal cancers remains poor because:
    a. The disease is usually local in nature.
    b. Diagnostic procedures do not exist for this disease.
    c. Most tumors are radioresistant.
    d. The majority of esophageal cancers are diagnosed late.

5. In esophageal cancer, two of the signs on physical examination include ptosis of the eyelid and miotic pupils. These signs are collectively called:
    a. Turner's syndrome.
    b. Jenny's syndrome.
    c. Horner's syndrome.
    d. En bloc syndrome.

6. The major postoperative complication associated with esophageal cancer is:
    a. Wound-healing problems.
    b. Dysphagia.
    c. Myelosuppression.
    d. Respiratory arrest.

7. Side effects from radiation therapy for esophageal cancer include:
    a. Diarrhea.
    b. Pulmonary emboli.
    c. Neurotoxicity.
    d. Dysphagia.

8. Screening for gastric cancer includes the diagnostic procedure(s) of:
    a. Abdominal chest radiographs.
    b. Serum hemoglobin values.
    c. Double-contrast barium studies with upper gastrointestinal endoscopy.
    d. Colonoscopy with colonic lavage.

9. What type of nutritional feeding route would be used for someone with gastric cancer?
   a. Nasogastric (NG) tube.
   b. Jejunostomy.
   c. Percutaneous enteral gastric (PEG) tube.
   d. Gastric tube (G-tube).

10. The most common chemotherapeutic agent used in treating gastric cancer is:
    a. Ifosphamide.
    b. 5-fluorouracil (5-FU).
    c. Prednisone.
    d. Thiotepa.

11. The name of the surgical procedure in which the entire stomach is removed along with lymph nodes and the first portion of the duodenum, is called a:
    a. Total gastrectomy.
    b. Billroth I subtotal resection.
    c. Gastroduodenostomy.
    d. En-bloc gastric dissection.

12. A diet low in fat, low in protein, and high in nitrate and smoked and salted foods are risk factors for what type of cancer?
    a. Rectal.
    b. Breast.
    c. Gastric.
    d. Esophageal.

13. Which of the following infections is a risk factor for gastric cancer?
    a. *Staphylococcus aureus.*
    b. *Klebsiella* species.
    c. *Helicobacter pylori.*
    d. *Chlamydia* species.

14. Anatomically, the sigmoid colon is between the:
    a. Rectum and descending colon.
    b. Transverse colon and descending colon.
    c. Cecum and hepatic flexture.
    d. Ascending colon and transverse colon.

15. The absorption of water and electrolytes occurs predominantly in what part of the colon?
    a. Ascending.
    b. Descending.
    c. Sigmoid.
    d. Rectum.

16. One of the signs for colorectal cancer is partial bowel obstruction. The stool during a partial bowel obstruction looks:
    a. Completely formed but hard.
    b. Watery.
    c. Normal.
    d. Pencil-shaped.

17. Which of the following antigens is used to monitor the response of therapy in colorectal cancer?
    a. Alpha-fetoprotein (AFP).
    b. Tumor necrosis factor (TNF).
    c. Carcinoembryonic antigen (CEA).
    d. Oncofetal protein (OFP).

18. For which of the following diagnostic tests do you refrain from eating red meat, poultry, fish, horseradish, turnips, and beets for 72 hours before the test?
    a. Computer axial tomography (CAT) scan.
    b. Stool for occult blood.
    c. Positron emission tomography (PET) scan.
    d. Electroencephalogram (EEG).

19. The primary treatment for the majority of persons with colorectal cancer is:
    a. Surgery.
    b. Chemotherapy.
    c. Radiation therapy.
    d. Immunotherapy.

20. Treatment for cancer of the anus usually results in what type of ostomy?
    a. Ileostomy.
    b. Colostomy.
    c. Ileal conduit.
    d. No ostomy results from treatment.

21. Which of the following is a genetic risk factor for colorectal cancers?
    a. Fanconi's anemia.
    b. History of rheumatoid arthritis.
    c. Low-fat, high-fiber diet.
    d. Familial polyposis.

22. Which of the following types of diet would increase transit time in the colon, thereby allowing more time for interaction of stool with the mucosa?
    a. High-protein.
    b. High-fat.
    c. Low-fiber.
    d. High-fiber.

23. If a client with a colostomy is taking bismuth subgallate (Derifill), 250 mg PO, qid, what problem related to the colostomy are they trying to manage?
    a. Skin irritation.
    b. Folliculitis.
    c. Fecal odor.
    d. Candidiasis.

*24. Eight hours after having surgery for colon cancer, a client's vital signs 2 hours previously were: pulse, 78; respirations, 18; blood pressure, 126/74 mm Hg. Currently, his vital signs are: pulse, 90; respirations, 20; blood pressure, 80/60 mm Hg. The most likely cause of the changes in vital signs is:
    a. Paralytic ileus.
    b. Infection.
    c. Protrusion of stoma onto abdomen.
    d. Bleeding.

* Reflects advanced oncology nursing content

*25. Upon routine colonoscopy at age 52, your client had a polyp excised in the transverse colon that pathology determined to be a villous adenoma. Your knowledge concerning these facts leads you to recommend what type of follow-up to the client?
   a.   Yearly stool examination for occult blood.
   b.   Yearly colonoscopy.
   c.   Yearly sigmoidoscopy.
   d.   Eat a high-fiber, low-fat diet.

*26. If surgical margins are positive for cancer of the colon, the recommended treatment is:
   a.   Further surgery.
   b.   Preoperative radiation followed by surgery.
   c.   Postoperative radiation therapy.
   d.   Chemotherapy followed by bone marrow transplant.

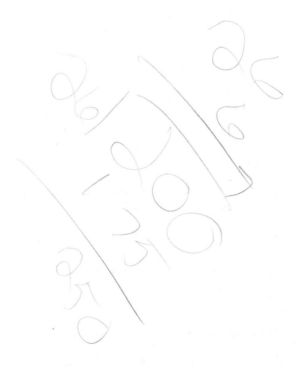

ANSWERS

1. **(c)**   Esophageal cancer is often systemic at diagnosis, with 20% of individuals presenting with a second primary and with most having lymph node involvement.

2. **(d)**   Forced expiratory volume of at least 70% is recommended before a client undergoes surgery for esophageal cancer.

3. **(a)**   Current treatments for esophageal cancer include combination chemotherapy (5-FU, cisplatin, and mitomycin-C, usually) with radiation therapy.

4. **(d)**   The prognosis for esophageal cancers is poor because most are diagnosed at late stages.

5. **(c)**   Horner's syndrome is ptosis of the eyelid with miotic pupils. This is one of the assessments to do during a workup for esophageal cancer.

6. **(a)**   Postoperative complications for esophageal cancer include impaired wound healing, aspiration, ARDS, and anastomotic leak.

7. **(d)**   Radiation side effects in esophageal cancer treatment include fatigue, nausea, dysphagia, fistula, and vomiting and myelosuppression with combined therapies.

8. **(c)**   Screening for gastric cancer, which has a high incidence in Japan, includes the use of double-contrast barium studies with upper gastrointestinal endoscopy.

9. **(b)**   A jejunostomy feeding is appropriate for someone with gastric cancer.

10. **(b)**   The most common chemotherapy agent used to treat gastric cancer is 5-fluorouracil (5-FU). Other agents include adriamycin, platinol, mitomycin-C, MTX, and etoposide.

11. **(a)**   A total gastrectomy is a surgical procedure in which the entire stomach, lymph nodes, and a portion of the duodenum are removed owing to gastric cancer.

12. **(c)**   Dietary risk factors for gastric cancer include low-fat, low-protein diets; salted meat and fish; low consumption of vitamins A and C; smoked foods; and nitrate-containing foods.

13. **(c)**   *Helicobacter pylori* infection is a risk factor for gastric cancer.

14. **(a)**   The sigmoid colon is between the descending colon and rectum.

15. **(a)**   The absorption of water and electrolytes occurs mostly in the ascending colon.

16. **(d)**   Partial bowel obstruction elicits pencil-shaped stool, which is a sign of colorectal cancer.

17. **(c)**   Carcinoembryonic antigen (CEA) is used to monitor therapeutic treatment response in colorectal cancers.

18. **(b)**   Before the diagnostic test of stool for occult blood, the client should refrain from eating the following foods for 72 hours: red meat, poultry, fish, horseradish, turnips, and beets.

19. **(a)**   Surgery is the primary treatment modality for colorectal cancer.

20. **(b)**   A colostomy usually results from treatment employed for cancer of the anus.

21. (d) Familial polyposis, Gardner's syndrome, Turcot syndrome, and juvenile polyposis are genetic risk factors for colorectal cancers.

22. (c) A low-fiber diet increases transit time in the colon, allowing more time for carcinogens in the stool to interact with the mucosa.

23. (c) Bismuth subgallate (Derifill) are medications used to manage fecal odor or problems in persons with a colostomy.

*24. (d) Symptoms of bleeding after surgery for colorectal cancer include changes in blood pressure, heart rate, and respiration along with increased wound drainage.

*25. (b) Villous adenomas are polyps that are likely to become malignant, so routine follow-up care includes a yearly colonoscopy.

*26. (c) If examination of surgical margins is positive for cancer cells in patients with colorectal cancer, the treatment of choice is postoperative radiation therapy.

* Reflects advanced oncology nursing content

CHAPTER 26

Nursing Care of the Client with Leukemia

QUESTIONS

1. Which of the following blood-forming organs are responsible for developing immunity and transporting carbon dioxide, hemoglobin, and oxygen?
   a. Bone marrow.
   b. Liver.
   c. Spleen.
   d. Thyroid gland.

2. The most common form of leukemia in children is:
   a. Chronic lymphatic.
   b. Chronic promyelocytic.
   c. Acute myelogenous.
   d. Acute lymphocytic.

3. When chemotherapy is administered into the central nervous system to treat leukemia, it is called:
   a. Intrathecal chemotherapy.
   b. Systemic chemotherapy.
   c. Intracavitary chemotherapy.
   d. Blastic chemotherapy.

4. On educating a client and family about treatment for leukemia, you teach that the initial chemotherapy will be given in high doses in hope of eradicating the leukemia. The name for this initial treatment phase is:
   a. Initiation.
   b. Induction.
   c. Intensification.
   d. Consolidation.

5. Chemotherapy in children with leukemia is generally continued for how long?
   a. Days.
   b. Weeks.
   c. Months.
   d. Years.

6. If relapse occurs in a child with acute lymphocyte leukemia, the next treatment of choice would be:
   a. Radiation therapy alone.
   b. Surgery alone.
   c. Bone marrow transplant.
   d. Chemotherapy alone.

7. What musculoskeletal physical symptoms would you find in a newly diagnosed leukemia patient?
   a. Papilledema.
   b. Joint pain.
   c. Ecchymoses.
   d. Pale mucous membranes.

8. In a person diagnosed with leukemia, what laboratory result would be abnormal?
   a. Vitamin A.
   b. Creatine phosphokinase.
   c. Blood urea nitrogen.
   d. Differential leukocyte count.

9. Routine follow-up care for a client with leukemia would include what diagnostic procedure?
   a. Bronchoscopy.
   b. Cystoscopy.
   c. Colposcopy.
   d. Bone marrow biopsy.

10. Which of the following conditions is a precursor to septic shock in the person with leukemia?
    a. Disseminated intravascular coagulation (DIC).
    b. Myelosuppression.
    c. Mucositis.
    d. Tumor lysis syndrome (TLS).

11. The most common complication of leukostasis in a person with leukemia is:
    a. Cardiac dysrhythmias.
    b. Splenomegaly.
    c. Cerebral hemorrhage.
    d. Renal failure.

*12. A 58-year-old client is diagnosed with chronic lymphocytic leukemia. You note that the client has immune-mediated cytopenia that needs to be controlled. The most appropriate medication to control this is:
    a. Mannitol.
    b. Granulocyte colony-stimulating factor.
    c. Prednisone.
    d. Vitamin E.

---

* Reflects advanced oncology nursing content

ANSWERS

1. (a)   The bone marrow is a blood-forming organ responsible for developing immunity, maintaining hemostasis, and transporting carbon dioxide, hemoglobin, and oxygen.

2. (d)   Acute lymphocytic leukemia is the most common type of childhood leukemia.

3. (a)   Intrathecal is the term used to denote chemotherapy administered into the central nervous system.

4. (b)   Induction is the term applied to initial high-dose chemotherapy in the leukemia patient to eradicate all leukemic cells.

5. (d)   Chemotherapy for children with leukemia is generally continued for years, including a postremission therapy time of 2 to 3 years.

6. (c)   Bone marrow transplant is the treatment of choice for relapsed acute lymphocytic leukemia in children.

7. (b)   Joint pain and inflammation of the joints are musculoskeletal signs during physical examination that are indicative of leukemia.

8. (d)   Abnormal lab values in leukemia include the differential leukocyte count, uric acid, liver function tests, platelet count, and red blood cell count.

9. (d)   Routine follow-up diagnostic care for leukemic clients include bone marrow biopsies and lumbar punctures.

10. (b)   Myelosuppression is a precursor to septic shock.

11. (c)   Leukostasis increases blood viscosity as well as intracranial pressure, causing thrombi and cerebral or pulmonary hemorrhage.

*12. (c)   Prednisone is the drug of choice to treat immune-related cytopenia in CLL.

---

* Reflects advanced oncology nursing content

CHAPTER 27

Nursing Care of Clients with Lymphoma and Multiple Myeloma

QUESTIONS

1. The malignant cell of Hodgkin's disease is called:
   a. Philadelphia chromosome.
   b. Reed-Sternberg cell.
   c. Herpes papillomavirus (HPV) cell.
   d. Burkitt's cell.

2. The classic clinical presentation of a person with Hodgkin's disease is a person with:
   a. Enlarged lymph nodes.
   b. Hemoptysis.
   c. Diaphoresis.
   d. Weight gain.

3. Which of the following is TRUE about non-Hodgkin's lymphomas (lymphocytic lymphomas)?
   a. Most are T-cell malignancies.
   b. Usually diagnosed in a single lymph node.
   c. A nonaggressive, localized malignancy.
   d. Involvement of the bone marrow is common.

4. Which neoplastic disease produces high blood levels of monoclonal immunoglobulins, or M proteins?
   a. Malignant melanoma.
   b. Monocytic leukemia.
   c. Multiple myeloma.
   d. Squamous cell carcinoma of the lung.

5. The main organ affected by hypercalcemia and hyperviscosity in multiple myeloma is the:
   a. Kidney.
   b. Lung.
   c. Bone marrow.
   d. Heart.

6. The laboratory test used to diagnose multiple myeloma is:
   a. Red blood cell count.
   b. Urine pH level.
   c. Serum protein electrophoresis.
   d. Serum creatinine level.

7. An 18-year-old man comes to the clinic with the following symptoms: enlarged supraclavicular and cervical lymph nodes, temperature 101° F orally, night sweats, and a 4-pound weight loss in the past 5 days. These are symptoms of what neoplastic disease?
   a. Malignant melanoma.
   b. Hodgkin's disease.
   c. Non-Hodgkin's lymphoma.
   d. Chronic lymphocytic leukemia.

*8. Your client is diagnosed with lymphoma and multiple mediastinal disease. He has red conjunctivae and shortness of breath. The client is at high risk for what oncologic emergency?
   a. Tumor lysis syndrome.
   b. Superior vena cava syndrome.
   c. Hypercalcemia.
   d. Pulmonary embolism.

* Reflects advanced oncology nursing content

ANSWERS

1. **(b)**   The Reed-Sternberg cell is the malignant cell of Hodgkin's disease.

2. **(a)**   The classic presentation of a person with Hodgkin's disease includes enlarged lymph nodes, fever, weight loss, and night sweats.

3. **(d)**   Non-Hodgkin's lymphoma is a B-cell, sometimes T-cell, malignancy that usually presents with disseminated disease, including involvement of the marrow and liver.

4. **(c)**   Multiple myeloma is a plasma cell malignancy that produces monoclonal immunoglobulins, called M proteins.

5. **(a)**   Multiple myeloma affects the kidneys by means of amyloid deposits, hypercalcemia, or hyperviscosity.

6. **(c)**   Multiple myeloma is diagnosed by bone marrow biopsy, serum protein electrophoresis, or urine immunoelectrophoresis.

7. **(b)**   Symptoms of Hodgkin's disease include cervical, mediastinal, or supraclavicular lymph node enlargement; fever; anorexia; night sweats; shortness of breath (SOB); weakness; weight loss; bone pain; and urinary changes.

*8. **(b)**   Clients with lymphoma and Hodgkin's disease with mediastinal disease are at high risk for superior vena cava syndrome (SVCS). Red conjunctivae and SOB are signs of SVCS.

* Reflects advanced oncology nursing content

CHAPTER 28

Nursing Care of the Client with Bone and Soft-Tissue Cancers

QUESTIONS

1. Most soft-tissue sarcomas appear in what part of the body?
   a. Lower extremities.
   b. Upper extremities.
   c. Central nervous system.
   d. Oral cavity.

2. Which one of the following is a common reconstruction method for bone cancers?
   a. Autografts.
   b. Allografts.
   c. Neoadjuvant chemotherapy.
   d. Thoracotomy.

3. Which of the following statements is TRUE about phantom limb pain or sensation after amputation for bone cancer?
   a. Usually takes 5 to 10 years to resolve.
   b. Client's main concern is fear of hemorrhage.
   c. Usually increased with diet high in nitrates.
   d. Greater when amputation site is more proximal.

4. The primary nursing diagnosis associated with persons treated for bone neoplasms is:
   a. Body image disturbance.
   b. Ineffective denial.
   c. Impaired skin integrity.
   d. Activity intolerance.

5. Physical examination of an osteosarcoma reveals that the mass feels:
   a. Firm, nontender, warm.
   b. Firm, tender, cool.
   c. Soft, painful, cool.
   d. Soft, nontender, warm.

6. Preoperative teaching for bone cancers should include information on what allied health service?
   a. Cardiac rehabilitation.
   b. Dental hygiene.
   c. Physical therapy.
   d. Enterostomal therapy.

*7. An aggressive sarcoma has what type of appearance on a radiograph?
   a. Geographic.
   b. Moth-eaten.
   c. Water-bottle.
   d. Striped flag.

---

* Reflects advanced oncology nursing content

ANSWERS

1. **(a)**   Soft-tissue sarcomas occur most often in the trunk and lower extremities.

2. **(b)**   Allografts of bones, tendons, or ligaments are commonly used in reconstruction for bone cancers.

3. **(d)**   Phantom limb pain or sensation is greater if the amputation is more proximal and usually take a few months to resolve. Sensations include itching, tingling, pressure, and burning pain.

4. **(d)**   The primary nursing diagnosis for persons with bone cancer is activity intolerance.

5. **(a)**   Osteosarcomas feel firm, nontender, and warm. Pain is usually a late sign and is worse at night.

6. **(c)**   Physical therapy is the allied health service that needs to be included in preoperative teaching of persons with bone cancers.

*7. **(b)**   Moth-eaten and permeative are the terms used to describe radiographic appearances of aggressive sarcomas.

* Reflects advanced oncology nursing content

CHAPTER 29

Nursing Care of the Client with HIV-Related Cancer

QUESTIONS

1. Human immunodeficiency virus (HIV) binds to T4 cells. What type of cell is a T4 cell?
   a. Erythrocyte.
   b. Thrombocyte.
   c. Stem cell.
   d. Lymphocyte.

2. What is the most frequent malignant disease found in persons infected with the human immunodeficiency virus (HIV)?
   a. Osteosarcoma.
   b. Colon cancer.
   c. B-cell lymphoma.
   d. Multiple myeloma.

3. Human immunodeficiency virus (HIV)–related Kaposi's sarcoma has skin lesions of what color?
   a. Green.
   b. Blue.
   c. Purple.
   d. Yellow.

4. Signs of decreased attention span, personality change, and generalized seizures are associated with what system metastasis for HIV-infected persons?
   a. Gastrointestinal (GI) system.
   b. Central nervous system (CNS).
   c. Bone marrow.
   d. Reticuloendothelial system.

5. The enzyme-linked immunosorbent assay (ELISA) used for screening for HIV (human immunodeficiency virus) requires what type of sample?
   a. Blood.
   b. Urine.
   c. Sputum.
   d. Bone marrow.

6. Which of the following treatment modalities are generally NOT used with HIV-related lymphoma?
   a. Biologic response modifiers.
   b. Chemotherapy.
   c. Radiation therapy.
   d. Surgery.

7. HIV-related lymphoma is treated with:
   a. Combination chemotherapy.
   b. Vinca alkaloid therapy only.
   c. Surgery.
   d. Brachytherapy and biologic response modifiers.

8. Persons with HIV-related Kaposi's sarcoma have the worst prognosis when they have:
   a. Infection(s).
   b. Diarrhea.
   c. Malnutrition.
   d. Rigors.

9. Children born to mothers who are HIV-infected have a greater chance of being HIV-positive if the mother:
   a. Ceases sexual activity.
   b. Refuses blood products.
   c. Refuses prenatal antiretroviral therapy.
   d. Continues to use needles for insulin injections.

10. Persons with Kaposi's sarcoma can experience obstruction of lymph flow from the sarcoma's growth. This causes:
    a. Increased cardiac output.
    b. Anasarca.
    c. Hypertension.
    d. Lymphedema.

11. Laboratory results of viral load in persons with HIV indicate the amount of virus in the:
    a. Central nervous system.
    b. Lymphatic system.
    c. Blood.
    d. Reticuloendothelial system.

12. The primary nursing diagnosis for persons with HIV is:
    a. Fatigue.
    b. Risk for infection.
    c. Altered nutrition; less than body requirements.
    d. Altered thought processes.

13. Standard precautions (universal precautions) do NOT apply to which body fluids:
    a. Semen.
    b. Cerebrospinal fluid.
    c. Urine.
    d. Blood.

*14. Human immunodeficiency virus (HIV)–infected women have a more rapid progression of what type of cancer compared with noninfected women?
    a. Cervical cancer.
    b. Ovarian cancer.
    c. Rectal cancer.
    d. Head and neck cancer.

* Reflects advanced oncology nursing content

ANSWERS

1. **(d)**   A T4 cell is a type of lymphocyte.

2. **(c)**   B-cell lymphoma and Kaposi's sarcoma are common malignancies found in persons with HIV infection.

3. **(c)**   HIV-related Kaposi's sarcoma skin lesions are pink to purple in color.

4. **(b)**   CNS metastasis from HIV infection includes signs of headache, neurologic deficits, seizures, memory loss, decreased attention span, personality change, and cognitive dysfunctions.

5. **(a)**   The ELISA test used in screening persons for HIV infection requires a blood sample.

6. **(d)**   Surgery is generally not used to treat HIV-related lymphoma, unless lesions interfere with function.

7. **(a)**   Combination chemotherapy (i.e., M-BACOD) is common treatment for HIV-related lymphoma.

8. **(a)**   Persons with HIV-related Kaposi's sarcoma have the worst prognosis—less than 1 year—if they have a major infection.

9. **(c)**   Children have a 30% to 50% chance of being infected with HIV if their mother refuses prenatal antiretroviral therapy.

10. **(d)**   Obstruction of lymph flow from Kaposi's sarcoma causes lymphedema.

11. **(c)**   Viral load laboratory results in HIV-infected persons indicate the amount of virus in the blood only, not amounts in the CNS or lymphatic system.

12. **(b)**   Risk for infection is the primary nursing diagnosis for persons with HIV infection.

13. **(c)**   Standard precautions do NOT apply to urine, vomitus, tears, saliva, nasal secretions, perspiration, or feces, unless they contain blood, according to the CDC.

*14. **(a)**   HIV-infected women have an increased risk for cervical cancer proliferation and require teaching.

* Reflects advanced oncology nursing content

30

Nursing Care of the Client with Genital Cancer

QUESTIONS

1. The majority of invasive cervical carcinomas arise from what anatomic body part?
   a. Vagina.
   b. Ovary.
   c. Endocervix.
   d. Squamocolumnar junction.

2. The virus associated with cervical carcinoma is:
   a. Epstein-Barr virus (EBV).
   b. Human papillomavirus (HPV).
   c. *Chlamydia* virus.
   d. Cytomegalovirus (CMV).

3. When should Papanicolaou (Pap) smears be initiated?
   a. Age 16 years.
   b. 1 month after beginning of menses.
   c. After first pregnancy.
   d. At initiation of sexual intercourse.

4. Screening procedures for cancer of the cervix include the Papanicolaou (Pap) smear and:
   a. Bimanual pelvic examination.
   b. Colposcopy.
   c. Cone biopsy.
   d. Cervical biopsy.

5. Which of the following decision-making processes is correct for possible cervical cancer?
   a. Endocervical curettage, positive results on Pap (Papanicolaou) smear, cone biopsy.
   b. Negative results on Pap smear, repeat if negative results, abnormal results on colposcopy.
   c. Positive results on Pap smear, cervical biopsy, colposcopy results abnormal.
   d. Positive results on Pap smear, colposcopy results abnormal, cervical biopsy.

6. Evaluation of the extent of cervical cancer and whether there is regional lymph node metastasis is best accomplished by use of what diagnostic test?
   a. Computed tomographic scan (CT).
   b. Cystoscopy.
   c. Intravenous pyelogram (IVP).
   d. Lymphangiography.

7. A 29-year-old woman has cervical carcinoma and has chosen radiation therapy as her treatment option. What type of radiation will she receive?
   a. Teletherapy.
   b. Brachytherapy.
   c. Cone therapy.
   d. Ultraviolet.

8. The primary surgical treatment for early stage cervical cancer is a:
   a. Unilateral salpingo-oophorectomy.
   b. Endocervical conization.
   c. Radical hysterectomy.
   d. Paraaortic lymph node dissection.

9. Treatment of recurrent local disease of cervical carcinoma includes surgery composed of a radical hysterectomy, pelvic lymph node dissection, removal of bladder or rectosigmoid colon, and creation of an ileal conduit or colostomy. This surgery is known as:
   a. Radical invasive hysterectomy.
   b. Pelvic exenteration.
   c. Extrapelvic disseminated excision (EDE).
   d. Total pelvic lymphadenectomy.

10. A 24-year-old woman reports the following health history: history of herpes simplex virus, type 2, and human papillomavirus infection; first sexual intercourse at age 15, with 44 partners since age 15; smoked 2 packs of cigarettes per day for 8 years; constipation; rectal bleeding; and pelvic flank pain. These are risk factors and signs or symptoms of what type of cancer?
   a. Ovarian.
   b. Colon.
   c. Cervix.
   d. Lung.

11. Anatomically, the endometrium is part of the:
   a. Uterus.
   b. Vagina.
   c. Cervix.
   d. Ovaries.

12. The cause of endometrial cancer is thought to be:
   a. Cigarette smoking.
   b. Multiple sexual partners.
   c. Endogenous estrogens.
   d. Endogenous progesterones.

13. In staging endometrial cancer, it must be determined whether there is bladder involvement. This is determined by:
   a. Barium enema.
   b. Sigmoidoscopy.
   c. Positron emission tomography (PET) scan.
   d. Cystoscopy.

14. Preinvasive endometrial cancer is treated with:
   a. Progesterone.
   b. Estrogen.
   c. Brachytherapy.
   d. Combination chemotherapy.

15. What lifestyle changes can modify the risks of endometrial cancer?
   a. Maintain ideal body weight.
   b. Take calcium supplements daily.
   c. Avoid constipation.
   d. Maintain abstinence from sexual intercourse.

16. To prevent postoperative venous stasis you should teach the client to:
   a. Avoid the use of the knee gatch in bed.
   b. Remain still in bed.
   c. Remove antiembolic stocking after getting out of bed.
   d. Avoid ambulation.

17. The spread of ovarian cancer usually occurs to what organ?
    a. Spleen.
    b. Rectum.
    c. Lungs.
    d. Brain.

18. What serum antigen study is done to help diagnose and monitor ovarian carcinoma?
    a. CEA.
    b. AFP.
    c. CA-125.
    d. Beta human chorionic gonadotropin (β-hCG).

19. A "second-look" surgical procedure in patients with ovarian cancer is done to:
    a. Remove tumor missed by the original surgery.
    b. Determine if there is bladder involvement.
    c. Evaluate the response to chemotherapy.
    d. Explore lymph node involvement.

20. For which one of the following cancers would chemotherapy be given intraperitoneally?
    a. Colon.
    b. Lymphoma.
    c. Myeloma.
    d. Ovarian.

21. First-line adjuvant chemotherapy to treat ovarian cancer consists of:
    a. Interleukin-2 only.
    b. 5-FU only.
    c. Paclitaxel and cisplatin.
    d. Cyclophosphamide and methotrexate.

22. The main treatment modality used for vulvar cancer is:
    a. Chemotherapy.
    b. Radiation therapy.
    c. Biologic response modifier therapy.
    d. Surgery.

23. The primary nursing diagnosis for female genital cancers is:
    a. Body image disturbance.
    b. Ineffective individual coping.
    c. Grieving.
    d. Constipation.

24. If pelvic lymph node dissection is completed as part of surgical treatment for metastatic ovarian cancer, what would you teach the client to monitor for?
    a. Leg edema.
    b. Constipation.
    c. Abdominal distention.
    d. Flank pain.

25. Anatomically, the vagina is between the:
    a. Hilar lymph nodes and ovaries.
    b. Uterus and vulva.
    c. Corpus and sigmoid colon.
    d. Endocervix and ectocervix.

26. Which of the following cancers is considered curable?
- a. Vaginal.
- b. Testicular.
- c. Lung.
- d. Breast.

*27. A 60-year-old woman has a history of infertility, nulliparity, obesity, diabetes, and hypertension. These factors place her at great risk for what type of cancer?
- a. Ovarian.
- b. Cervical.
- c. Endometrial.
- d. Colon.

*28. You suspect a client to have nonseminoma germ-cell testicular tumor (NSGCTT). Your assessment to verify this should include:
- a. Abdominal CT scan and CA-125 marker.
- b. Lymph node examination with serum AFP marker.
- c. Testicular exam and proctosigmoidoscopy.
- d. Chest x-ray and intravenous pyelogram (IVP).

*29. A 66-year-old man is about to undergo a total penectomy for cancer of the penis. Your preoperative teaching should include a discussion about what type of ostomy?
- a. Jejunostomy.
- b. Ascending colostomy.
- c. Descending colostomy.
- d. Urostomy.

---

* Reflects advanced oncology nursing content

ANSWERS

1. **(d)** Most invasive carcinomas of the cervix arise from the squamocolumnar junction.

2. **(b)** Human papillomavirus (HPV) is associated with cancer of the cervix.

3. **(d)** Pap smears should be started at the initiation of sexual intercourse or age 18, whichever is first.

4. **(a)** Screening procedures for cancer of the cervix include a Pap smear and bimanual pelvic examination.

5. **(d)** The proper decision-making process for possible cancer of the cervix is to follow a positive (abnormal) PAP smear with examination of the cervix under magnification by use of a colposcope and then a cervical biopsy if colposcopy reveals abnormalities.

6. **(a)** Evaluation of the extent of cervical cancer and possible lymph node metastases is best accomplished by a CT or MRI scan.

7. **(b)** Intracavitary brachytherapy implants are a radiation treatment option for cancer of the cervix.

8. **(c)** A radical hysterectomy is the surgical treatment for early-stage cancer of the cervix. For women over 40, a bilateral salpingo-oophorectomy is also done.

9. **(b)** A pelvic exenteration is the term used for the surgical procedures applied to treat recurrent local cervical cancer. It includes a radical hysterectomy, pelvic lymph node dissection, and removal of bladder with ileal conduit or removal of rectosigmoid colon with colostomy.

10. **(c)** Cervical cancer risk factors are: smoking, early intercourse, multiple partners, HIV or herpes simplex 2 virus infection, immunosuppression, and symptoms of urinary or colon and pelvic pain.

11. **(a)** The endometrium is the inner layer of three layers of the uterus.

12. **(c)** Endogenous estrogens are thought to be the cause of endometrial cancer.

13. **(d)** Cystoscopy is done to determine bladder involvement from endometrial cancer.

14. **(a)** Preinvasive endometrial cancer is treated with simple hysterectomy or progesterone administration.

15. **(a)** To modify the risks of endometrial cancer, educate the client to maintain ideal body weight and, if postmenopausal with uterus, suggest estrogen plus progesterone hormone replacement therapy.

16. **(a)** To prevent postoperative venous stasis, teach the client to ambulate, turn in bed, do isometric leg exercises, use antiembolic stockings, and avoid the use of the knee gatch in the bed.

17. **(c)** The spread of ovarian cancer is most common to the liver and lungs.

18. **(c)** CA-125 is an antigen study used to diagnose and monitor ovarian cancer.

19. **(c)** A "second-look" procedure is a surgical procedure done after chemotherapy in ovarian cancer to evaluate the response to therapy. Approximately one-third of clients have evidence of disease on second-look surgery.

20. **(d)** Intraperitoneal chemotherapy is used to treat ovarian cancer.

21. **(c)** Adjuvant chemotherapy to treat ovarian cancer consists of paclitaxel and cisplatin or carboplatin. Additionally, recurrent disease is treated with cyclophosphamide, hexamethylmelamine, or hydroxyurea.

22. **(d)** Surgery is the main treatment modality for vulvar cancer.

23. **(a)** The primary nursing diagnosis for female genital cancer is body image disturbance followed by sexual dysfunction and ineffective coping.

24. **(a)** After lymph node dissection for ovarian cancer, the client should be taught to monitor for leg edema.

25. **(b)** Anatomically, the vagina is between the uterus and the vulva.

26. **(b)** Testicular cancer is one of the cancers considered curable. Others include thyroid, some cervical, and Hodgkin's disease.

*27. **(c)** Obesity, diabetes, and hypertension are a triad that places a female at risk for endometrial cancer. Peak age is 50 to 64, with high socioeconomic status and history of nulliparity, infertility, irregular menses, or Stein-Leventhal syndrome.

*28. **(b)** Nonseminoma germ-cell testicular tumors (NSGCTT) have a 65% chance of spread to the lymph nodes at diagnosis and positive serum results for AFP and β-hCG antigens.

*29. **(d)** A total penectomy includes the need for a perineal urostomy, so that urination may occur.

---

* Reflects advanced oncology nursing content

Nursing Care of the Client with Skin Cancer

QUESTIONS

1. Which of the following types of cancer is NOT a skin cancer?
   a. Myeloma.
   b. Melanoma.
   c. Basal cell.
   d. Squamous cell.

2. Which of the following is an early feature of a malignant melanoma lesion?
   a. Symmetrical.
   b. Color variegation.
   c. Diameter of less than 1 mm.
   d. Border is regular in appearance.

3. The diagnosis of skin cancers occurs by:
   a. Antigen studies.
   b. Biopsy.
   c. The measurement of diameter of the nodule.
   d. Endoscopic examination.

4. Surgical removal of nonmelanoma skin cancers by multiple progressive layers is known as:
   a. Mohs' surgery.
   b. Electrodesiccation.
   c. Curettage.
   d. Local excision.

5. The major risk factor for basal cell carcinoma is:
   a. Ultraviolet radiation over long periods.
   b. A few massive ultraviolet radiation burns from the sun.
   c. Long-term cigarette smoking.
   d. Dark natural hair color.

6. Persons with which of the following conditions are at risk for developing skin cancer?
   a. Chronic renal failure.
   b. Organ transplant recipient.
   c. Liver failure.
   d. Heroin addict.

7. When should sunscreen be reapplied to protect ourselves from ultraviolet radiation?
   a. Reapplication is not necessary.
   b. Every 8 hours.
   c. After swimming.
   d. When concurrently taking aspirin-containing products.

8. Dysplastic nevi are risk factors for what type of cancer?
   a. Retinoblastoma.
   b. Melanoma.
   c. Myeloma.
   d. Vulvar.

*9. A farmer has a 1-cm round skin nodule on his forehead that is shiny and translucent with a pearly hue. This is classic for:
     a. Padgett's disease.
     b. Melanoma.
     c. Basal cell carcinoma.
     d. Squamous cell carcinoma.

ANSWERS

1. **(a)** Myeloma is NOT a type of skin cancer but rather a malignant disease of plasma cells.

2. **(b)** Malignant melanoma has as its early symptoms irregular borders, asymmetry, color variegation, and lesions with a diameter of more than 6 mm.

3. **(b)** A definitive diagnosis for skin cancer occurs through biopsy results, either incisional or excisional.

4. **(a)** Mohs' surgical procedure is the removal of multiple tissue layers in a progressive manner until histology studies show tissue clear of nonmelanoma skin cancer cells.

5. **(a)** Ultraviolet radiation exposure over long periods, usually from the sun, is the major risk factor for basal cell carcinoma.

6. **(b)** Because of immunosuppression factors, persons who have received organ transplants are at high risk for developing skin cancers.

7. **(c)** Sunscreen should be reapplied every 2 to 3 hours and after swimming.

8. **(b)** Dysplastic nevi or atypical moles are risk factors for melanoma skin cancer.

*9. **(c)** Nodular basal cell carcinoma has the appearance of being shiny and translucent with a pearly hue.

---

* Reflects advanced oncology nursing content

CHAPTER 32

Nursing Care of the Client with Cancer of the Neurologic System

QUESTIONS

1. To obtain a cerebrospinal fluid sample from the brain you need to access the:
   a. Cerebrum.
   b. Thalamus.
   c. Ventricles.
   d. Meninges.

2. You have known your client with metastatic breast cancer for 4 years. She appears for a regular checkup and you note a lack of memory and personality changes. Her family says she has been extremely moody lately. These are signs of metastasis to what lobe of the brain?
   a. Frontal.
   b. Parietal.
   c. Occipital.
   d. Temporal.

3. Which of the following structures in the brain controls temperature?
   a. Cerebrum.
   b. Thalamus.
   c. Hypothalamus.
   d. Pons.

4. What characteristic of a headache would occur in someone with a brain tumor?
   a. Unilateral.
   b. Bilateral.
   c. Most severe when sleeping.
   d. Most severe after activity.

5. What is the most common solid tumor in children?
   a. Non-Hodgkin's lymphoma.
   b. Colon cancer.
   c. Hodgkin's disease.
   d. Brain cancer.

6. Which diagnostic test provides the best images of brain tumors?
   a. Computed tomography (CT) without contrast.
   b. Computed tomography (CT) with contrast.
   c. Magnetic resonance imaging (MRI) without contrast.
   d. Magnetic resonance imaging (MRI) with contrast.

7. When a brain tumor cannot be surgically resected, how is a tissue sample obtained from which to make a diagnosis?
   a. Stereotactic biopsy.
   b. Local excision.
   c. Cerebral angiogram.
   d. Bone marrow aspiration.

8. In the TNM classification, which of the indicators is most beneficial to persons with brain tumors?
   a. T: Tumor.
   b. N: Nodes.
   c. M: Metastasis.
   d. M: Multinodular.

9. Standard, conventional radiation therapy for primary brain tumors is given over what period of time?
   a. 3 days.
   b. 1 week.
   c. 6 to 7 weeks.
   d. 8 to 9 months.

10. Which of the following is a chemotherapeutic drug used to treat brain tumors because it crosses the blood-brain barrier?
    a. 5-Fluorouracil (5-FU).
    b. Methotrexate (MTX).
    c. Carmustine (BCNU).
    d. Cisplatin (Platinol, DDP).

11. Which part of a physical examination would be of primary importance in a person with a malignant glioma?
    a. Lymph nodes.
    b. Neurologic.
    c. Head and neck.
    d. Cardiovascular.

12. Steroids are often used in the treatment regimens for malignant brain tumors because steroids:
    a. Phagocytize malignant cells.
    b. Have a synergistic effect with vinca alkaloids.
    c. Increase blood pressure.
    d. Decrease cerebral edema.

13. Which of the following side effects is most likely a permanent result of radiation therapy for brain tumors?
    a. Pancytopenia.
    b. Personality dysfunction.
    c. Stomatitis.
    d. Alopecia.

14. Interventions of frequent rest periods and physical therapy to improve muscle tone are associated with which nursing diagnosis?
    a. Body image disturbance.
    b. Risk for activity intolerance.
    c. Risk for intracranial pressure increase.
    d. Altered family processes.

15. Loss of pituitary function caused by radiation therapy causes what physiologic result?
    a. Hyperglycemia.
    b. Increased osteoclastic activity.
    c. Leukocytosis.
    d. Loss of menstrual cycling.

16. A malignant tumor of the lumbar region of the spinal cord produces loss of function, beginning at the:
    a. Neck.
    b. Chest.
    c. Umbilicus.
    d. Hips.

17. Which of the following is an example of a motor dysfunction that may occur with a spinal cord tumor?
    a. Paresis of an arm.
    b. Numbness.
    c. Inability to differentiate hot and cold.
    d. Loss of sensation of touch.

*18. Your patient with lung cancer complains of being uncoordinated and losing balance. You know a CT of the brain is necessary. What part of the brain do you ask the radiologist to concentrate on in the evaluation?
    a. Temporal lobe.
    b. Cerebellum.
    c. Occipital lobe.
    d. Medulla oblongata.

*19. Your client has a history of a frontal lobe malignant tumor and a history of a temporal lobe malignant tumor. One year after treatment, on a routine office visit, you note irregularities in blood pressure, heartbeat, and respiration. This indicates a possible brain tumor in the:
    a. Hypothalamus.
    b. Cerebellum.
    c. Brainstem.
    d. Parietal lobe.

* Reflects advanced oncology nursing content

ANSWERS

1. **(c)** The ventricles of the brain are four connected cavities through which cerebrospinal fluid flows. The sample of CSF is accessed thru a ventriculostomy.

2. **(a)** Frontal lobe brain metastasis is responsible for personality changes, mood, memory, intellect, judgment, and abstract thinking.

3. **(c)** The hypothalamus is responsible for temperature, sleep, appetite, water balance, and blood pressure.

4. **(a)** Unilateral headaches, usually most severe on waking from sleep, are characteristic of a brain tumor.

5. **(d)** Brain tumors are the most common solid tumors in children.

6. **(d)** An MRI with contrast is the best diagnostic procedure to image the brain. The contrast enhances the tumor area.

7. **(a)** A stereotactic brain biopsy is done to obtain a sample of brain tissue from which a diagnosis can be made in persons with brain tumors that are unresectable.

8. **(a)** When using the TNM classification with brain tumors, only the tumor size is helpful, because node involvement is not applicable and metastasis outside the brain and nervous system is rare.

9. **(c)** Standard, conventional radiation therapy for primary brain tumors is usually given over 6 to 7 weeks.

10. **(c)** Nitrosoureas are commonly used to treat brain tumors because they cross the blood-brain barrier. Examples include carmustine (BCNU) and lomustine (CCNU).

11. **(b)** A neurologic examination is of primary importance in a person with a glioma, a malignant brain tumor.

12. **(d)** Steroids are used to treat brain tumors because they decrease cerebral edema.

13. **(d)** Alopecia will most likely be a permanent side effect from radiation for brain tumors.

14. **(b)** Physical therapy and frequent rest periods are associated with the nursing diagnosis of risk for activity intolerance.

15. **(d)** Loss of pituitary function resulting from radiation therapy causes a loss of menstrual cycling.

16. **(d)** A malignant tumor of the lumbar spine causes loss of function from the hips to the toes.

17. **(a)** Paresis of the arm is an example of a motor deficit. Sensory deficits include numbness, tingling, inability to distinguish hot from cold, and loss of touch or pain sensation.

*18. **(b)** The cerebellum is the portion of the brain responsible for balance and coordination.

*19. **(c)** Changes in blood pressure, heartbeat, or respiration may indicate a brain tumor in the brainstem.

* Reflects advanced oncology nursing content

33

Nursing Care of the Client with Head and Neck Cancer

QUESTIONS

1. Head and neck cancers usually metastasize to the:
   a. Colon.
   b. Brain.
   c. Lymphatics.
   d. Kidneys.

2. Most head and neck cancers originate in the:
   a. Sinuses.
   b. Oral cavity.
   c. Larynx.
   d. Nasopharynx.

3. Which of the following viruses is a risk factor for head and neck cancers?
   a. Herpes simplex.
   b. Human immunodeficiency virus (HIV).
   c. Hepatitis B.
   d. Human T-cell leukemia (HTCL).

4. A carcinoma found between the epiglottis and the cricoid cartilage would be a cancer of which anatomic site?
   a. Larynx.
   b. Nasopharynx.
   c. Oropharynx.
   d. Oral cavity.

5. On physical examination you note an enlarged lymph node 2 cm lateral from the chin. The node is best described as:
   a. Preauricular.
   b. Spinal accessory.
   c. Buccal.
   d. Submental.

6. Radiation therapy to the oropharynx causes xerostomia. Xerostomia is:
   a. Mouth sores.
   b. Decreased taste sensation.
   c. Decreased saliva production.
   d. Loss of speech.

7. Persistent hoarseness and throat pain are early symptoms of what type of head and neck cancer?
   a. Nose.
   b. Paranasal sinuses.
   c. Oral cavity.
   d. Larynx.

8. A potential side effect of a barium swallow x-ray examination is:
   a. Diarrhea.
   b. Anorexia.
   c. Pneumothorax.
   d. Constipation.

9. Which of the following diagnostic tests requires general anesthesia?
   a. Barium swallow.
   b. Panendoscopy.
   c. Cine-esophagography.
   d. Panoramic x-ray (Panorex).

10. Implanted iridium-192 or cesium-137 are used to treat malignant lesions of the tongue because these implants:
    a. Have fewer side effects than other implants.
    b. Are not radioactive.
    c. Can be implanted on an outpatient basis.
    d. Maximize radiation doses to the tumor.

11. You are assessing a suture line in a postoperative client with head and neck cancer and note that the suture line is red, indurated, and tender. These are signs of a possible:
    a. Fistula.
    b. Hemorrhage.
    c. Necrosis.
    d. Edema.

12. Monitoring renal function in persons receiving chemotherapy is best accomplished by obtaining a:
    a. 24-hour urine blood urea nitrogen/creatinine ratio.
    b. Serum sodium level.
    c. Serum creatinine level.
    d. pH of the urine.

13. Which of the following conditions may be a cause of fatigue?
    a. Thrombocytopenia.
    b. Anemia.
    c. Hypernatremia.
    d. Normovolemia.

14. Which of the following are risk factors for head and neck cancers?
    a. Multiple sexual partners.
    b. Work as a farmer.
    c. Low-fiber diet.
    d. Alcoholic beverage use.

15. A nursing intervention for a client who is receiving radiation therapy for head and neck cancer and has pruritus would be to:
    a. Apply hydrocortisone cream to the affected areas.
    b. Begin oral steroid therapy.
    c. Use potassium chloride compresses daily.
    d. Use saliva substitutes as needed.

16. What type of food would you recommend to a cancer patient who has altered oral mucous membranes?
    a. Regular.
    b. Low-fat, low-protein, high-roughage.
    c. High-roughage, high-protein.
    d. Soft, nonspicy, nonacidic.

17. Avoiding persons with colds, avoiding sharing eating utensils, and avoiding handling animal excreta are nursing interventions associated with what nursing diagnosis?
    a. Risk for injury.
    b. Risk of fluid volume deficit.
    c. Risk for infection.
    d. Altered oral mucous membranes.

18. In persons who have head and neck cancer, there should be a schedule of follow-up to detect recurrence or second primary tumors. During the first year, how often should follow-up be?
    a. Yearly.
    b. Every 6 months.
    c. Every 1 to 2 months.
    d. Weekly.

19. Which of the following pieces of equipment should NOT be kept at the bedside of a client with a tracheostomy?
    a. Inner cannula.
    b. Outer cannula.
    c. Tracheal dilator.
    d. Tongue depressor.

20. When is a noncuffed tracheostomy used in an adult?
    a. With mechanical ventilation.
    b. Risk of aspiration.
    c. After laryngectomy.
    d. When a fenestrated tube is in place.

21. The use of alcohol-containing mouthwashes are avoided for oral care of persons with head and neck cancer because alcohol:
    a. Is an illegal substance.
    b. Irritates the tissue, thereby increasing bleeding.
    c. Numbs the oral cavity.
    d. Dries the mucosa.

22. During neck dissection, the spinal accessory nerve and sternocleidomastoid muscle are resected. This causes:
    a. Shoulder droop.
    b. Scoliosis.
    c. Limited range of motion at the waist.
    d. Facial palsy.

23. Loss of the ability to perform the Valsalva maneuver predisposes clients to:
    a. Decreased intracranial pressure.
    b. Respiratory dysfunction.
    c. Constipation.
    d. Diarrhea.

24. During a carotid artery rupture of a person with a cuffed tracheostomy tube, in what position should the cuff be?
    a. Inflated.
    b. Deflated.
    c. Take out the tracheostomy tube altogether.
    d. Replace tracheostomy tube with obturator.

*25. Hyperoxygenation before and after suctioning in a person with a tracheostomy is necessary to prevent hypoxia and:
   a. Hypertension.
   b. Obstruction.
   c. Dysrhythmias.
   d. Aspiration.

*26. Aspiration is most likely to occur in which of the following clients?
   a. Post-supraglottic laryngectomy.
   b. Jejunostomy.
   c. Post-peritoneal shunt device surgery.
   d. After surgery for oral buccal squamous carcinoma.

*27. A client with a platelet count of less than 500/mm^3 and pulse rate of 92 becomes hypotensive, has a headache, and vomits once. Your major concern is that these are signs of:
   a. Sepsis.
   b. Hemorrhage.
   c. Cardiac tamponade.
   d. Pulmonary embolism.

* Reflects advanced oncology nursing content

ANSWERS

1. **(c)** Head and neck cancers usually metastasize via the neck to the lymphatics.

2. **(b)** Most head and neck cancers originate in the oral cavity.

3. **(a)** Viral risk factors for head and neck cancers include herpes simplex virus, human papillomavirus, and Epstein-Barr virus.

4. **(a)** Cancers of the larynx are found between the epiglottis and the cricoid cartilage.

5. **(d)** Submental lymph nodes are found near the area of the chin.

6. **(c)** Xerostomia is decreased saliva production, which is caused by radiation therapy to the oral cavity or oropharynx.

7. **(d)** Early symptoms of laryngeal cancer include hoarseness and throat pain.

8. **(d)** Constipation is a potential side effect from the use of barium in diagnostic tests.

9. **(b)** A panendoscopy is a surgical procedure in which a lighted scope is passed along the upper aerodigestive tract and biopsies are obtained. The procedure requires general anesthesia.

10. **(d)** Brachytherapy for cancer of the tongue is used because it maximizes radiation doses to the tumor.

11. **(a)** Suture lines that are red, indurated, and tender are signs of fistula development in postoperative head and neck cancer patients.

12. **(c)** Serum creatinine level is the best test for monitoring renal function in persons receiving chemotherapy.

13. **(b)** Anemia can be a cause of fatigue in persons with cancer.

14. **(d)** Using tobacco and drinking alcoholic beverages are risk factors for cancers of the head and neck.

15. **(a)** A nursing intervention for pruritus associated with radiation therapy is the application of a thin layer of hydrocortisone cream.

16. **(d)** Persons with altered oral mucous membranes should eat foods that are soft, nonspicy, and nonacidic.

17. **(c)** Risk for infection is the nursing diagnosis associated with the interventions of avoiding persons with colds and respiratory infections, avoiding sharing eating utensils and cups, and avoiding handling animal excreta.

18. **(c)** Follow-up for head and neck cancer should be every 1 to 2 months during the first year.

19. **(d)** A tongue depressor is not necessary at the bedside of a person with a tracheostomy. Necessary equipment includes a dilator, inner and outer cannulas, and scissors.

20. **(d)** Cuffed tracheostomies are used with respirators when there is risk of aspiration, and after laryngectomy. A fenestrated tube is used when the client can breathe without a cuffed tube.

21. **(d)** Avoid the use of alcohol-containing mouthwashes because alcohol dries the mucosa, leading to decreased humidification.

22. **(a)** In patients who have neck dissection in which the spinal accessory nerve and sternocleidomastoid muscle are resected, shoulder droop, some atrophy of the trapezius muscle, and forward spinal curvature are to be expected.

23. **(c)** Loss of the Valsalva maneuver predisposes persons to constipation; stool softeners are often prescribed for relief.

24. **(a)** A cuffed tracheostomy tube should always be inflated during a carotid artery rupture to prevent aspiration.

*25. **(c)** Hyperoxygenation before and after tracheal suctioning is done to prevent hypoxemia and dysrhythmias.

*26. **(a)** Patients who have post-supraglottic laryngectomies are at high risk for aspiration.

*27. **(b)** Hemorrhage that occurs during thrombocytopenia begins with a headache and usually hypotension, tachycardia, vomiting, and altered levels of consciousness follow.

---

* Reflects advanced oncology nursing content

CHAPTER 34

Nursing Implications
of Surgical Treatment

QUESTIONS

1. What is the name of the adjuvant surgical treatment used to reduce tumor volume to improve the effect of other cancer treatment modalities?
   a. Prophylactic surgery.
   b. Cytoreductive surgery.
   c. Palliative surgery.
   d. Salvage surgery.

2. Ulcerative colitis is an associated risk factor for what type of cancer?
   a. Stomach.
   b. Colon.
   c. Breast.
   d. Rectal.

3. Salvage therapy for cancer of the bladder includes what surgical approach?
   a. Abdominal-peritoneal resection.
   b. Ileostomy.
   c. Radical prostatectomy.
   d. Radical cystectomy.

4. Chemotherapy is administered to a client and, 3 weeks later, surgery is performed to remove the cancerous tumor. The surgery is known as what type of therapy?
   a. Primary.
   b. Conservative.
   c. Adjuvant.
   d. Salvage.

5. Which of the following is a therapeutic hardware device from which cerebrospinal fluid can be extracted?
   a. Gastrostomy tube.
   b. Ventricular reservoir.
   c. Arterial access catheter.
   d. Implantable insulin pump.

6. The use of liquid nitrogen to freeze tissue is called what type of surgery?
   a. Cryosurgery.
   b. Electrosurgery.
   c. Chemosurgery.
   d. Laser surgery.

7. A post-operative client is about to be discharged and you note that he or she lives on the third floor of an apartment building that has only stairs. The factor that influences your discharge planning would be:
   a. Self-care capabilities.
   b. Financial status.
   c. Home environment.
   d. Employment status.

8. Which of the following respiratory changes is associated with the aging process?
   a. Increased elasticity of lungs.
   b. Increased residual lung volume.
   c. Decreased ciliary action.
   d. Decreased glomerular filtration rate.

9. Which of the following serum laboratory tests is associated with nutritional assessment of a surgical patient?
   a. Prothrombin time.
   b. Electrolyte levels.
   c. Blood urea nitrogen level.
   d. Albumin level.

10. What type of dressing should be used in a post-operative client with copious drainage?
    a. Hydrocolloid.
    b. Occlusive, transparent, such as OpSite.
    c. Sugar and antacid mixture.
    d. Live yogurt with iodine gauze.

*11. Physiologic changes in the cardiovascular system associated with aging increased the potential for which post-operative complication?
    a. Atelectasis.
    b. Thrombosis with pulmonary emboli.
    c. Urinary tract infection.
    d. Hypovolemia.

* Reflects advanced oncology nursing content

ANSWERS

1. **(b)** Cytoreductive surgery reduces tumor volume to improve the effect of other cancer treatments.

2. **(b)** Ulcerative colitis is a risk factor for colon cancer.

3. **(d)** A radical cystectomy is salvage therapy for bladder cancer.

4. **(c)** Adjuvant therapy is therapy that is given after initial therapy or in conjunction with primary therapy.

5. **(b)** CSF can be extracted from a ventricular reservoir or ventriculostomy.

6. **(a)** Cryosurgery involves the use of liquid nitrogen to freeze tissue, thereby causing cellular death.

7. **(c)** Home environmental factors, such as living location, influences discharge planning.

8. **(c)** Respiratory changes associated with aging include decreased ciliary action, elasticity, forced expiratory volume, and residual lung volume.

9. **(d)** Nutritional assessment of a surgical patient is accomplished by assessing serum albumin levels.

10. **(a)** Copious drainage from a postsurgical client should be treated with hydrocolloid dressing or a collection device or bag.

*11. **(b)** Physiologic changes of the cardiovascular system associated with aging increase the potential postsurgical complications of shock, thrombosis, hypervolemia, decreased stress responses, and decreased wound healing.

* Reflects advanced oncology nursing content

CHAPTER 35

Nursing Implications of Radiation Therapy

QUESTIONS

1. Examples of radiation do *NOT* include:
   a. Heat.
   b. Water.
   c. Radiowaves.
   d. X-rays.

2. Electromagnetic radiation includes:
   a. X-rays.
   b. Electrons.
   c. Protons.
   d. Beta particles.

3. The most critical site for radiation damage is to affect cellular:
   a. RNA (ribonucleic acid).
   b. DNA (deoxyribonucleic acid).
   c. Nuclei.
   d. Chromatids.

4. Which of the following cells are most sensitive to the effects of radiation?
   a. Those in the resting phase.
   b. Nondividing.
   c. Slowly dividing.
   d. Rapidly dividing.

5. Dividing a dose of radiation into daily doses is known as dose:
   a. Response.
   b. Toleration.
   c. Fractionation.
   d. Amplification.

6. The aim of therapy in radiation therapy for the purpose of obtaining relief from superior vena cava syndrome is:
   a. Curative.
   b. Palliative.
   c. Control of the disease.
   d. Radioresistant.

7. Another name for external-beam radiation therapy is:
   a. Teletherapy.
   b. Brachytherapy.
   c. Radioimmunotherapy.
   d. Sealed source therapy.

8. The time it takes for 50% of radioactive atoms to decay is called:
   a. Particle lifetime (PLT).
   b. Half-life.
   c. Half-value.
   d. Disintegration decay time (DDT).

9. Which of the following is an unsealed radioactive source?
   a. Tracer dose source.
   b. Intracavity source.
   c. Interstitial source.
   d. Intraluminal source.

10. Which of the following teaching interventions is appropriate regarding persons wearing radiation dose or film badges?
    a. It is all right to wear someone else's badge just as long as you have a badge on.
    b. Wear the badge in a left shirt pocket so it is close to the heart.
    c. Wearing a film badge is optional.
    d. Badges are read and exchanged for a new one monthly.

11. The radiation-induced side effect of alopecia may occur if the client has radiation to the:
    a. Brain.
    b. Spine.
    c. Gastrointestinal tract.
    d. Bone marrow sites of the iliac crests.

12. An early side effect of radiation therapy to the large bowel is:
    a. Diarrhea.
    b. Constipation.
    c. Ileus.
    d. Xerostomia.

13. If a sealed radiation source is lost, who should be notified first?
    a. Emergency room physician on call.
    b. Nursing administrator.
    c. Radiation safety officer.
    d. Client's family.

*14. A client has a radioactive cesium-137 implant. If exposure is 40 mrem/hr at 3 feet, what would the exposure be at 6 feet?
    a. 80 mrem/hr.
    b. 6.6 mrem/hr.
    c. 20 mrem/hr.
    d. 10 mrem/hr.

*15. You are asked to teach a patient about tissue response to fractionation for teletherapy. You choose to teach about oxygenation and the cell cycle first. Which of the following statements would be true about oxygenation and the cell cycle?
    a. Hypoxic cells in the resting phase respond best to teletherapy.
    b. Well-oxygenated cells in mitosis respond best to teletherapy.
    c. Well-oxygenated cells in the resting phase respond best to teletherapy.
    d. Oxygen status and cell cycle have no effect associated with teletherapy.

* Reflects advanced oncology nursing content

ANSWERS

1. **(b)**   Water is not a type of radiation energy.

2. **(a)**   Electromagnetic radiation includes photons or gamma rays and x-rays.

3. **(b)**   Radiation is most critical when it affects cellular DNA.

4. **(d)**   The effects of radiation are greatest on rapidly dividing cells, such as those of the gastro-intestinal tract.

5. **(c)**   Dose fractionation is the term used to define dividing a dose of radiation into daily doses.

6. **(b)**   Palliative radiation therapy is meant to reduce symptoms, such as those from superior vena cava syndrome, spinal cord compression, or brain metastasis, and improve quality of life.

7. **(a)**   External-beam radiation therapy is also known as teletherapy.

8. **(b)**   Half-life is the term used to describe the time it takes for half of the radioactive atoms to decay.

9. **(a)**   Unsealed radioactive sources are radiopharmaceuticals that are tracer doses or therapeutic doses.

10. **(d)**   Wearing a radiation dose film badge includes only wearing your own, wearing it at waist level, and exchanging it monthly so the previous one can be read.

11. **(a)**   Radioactivity-induced alopecia occurs only if the client is radiated to the head for cancers such as brain cancer.

12. **(a)**   Diarrhea is an early side effect from radiation therapy to the large bowel.

13. **(c)**   If a sealed radiation source is lost, notify the radiation safety officer (RSO) first.

*14. **(d)**   Doubling distance to radiation exposure decreases the exposure to one-fourth of the original exposure received. Doubling the distance from 3 to 6 feet decreases the original exposure to one-fourth, or from 40 to 10 mrem/hr.

*15. **(b)**   Well-oxygenated tissues of cells in mitosis, which is followed by the G_2 phase, are more sensitive to teletherapy.

---

* Reflects advanced oncology nursing content

36

Nursing Implications of Biotherapy

QUESTIONS

1. Hematopoietic growth factors are classified as what type of agents?
   a. Biologic response modifiers.
   b. Chemotherapeutic.
   c. Immunodilutents.
   d. Monoclonal antibodies.

2. Interleukins are protein molecules responsible for communication between cells. Because interleukins are proteins, they fall under the generic term of:
   a. Monoclonal antibodies.
   b. Cytokines.
   c. Immunomodulators.
   d. Retinoids.

3. Use of retinoids should be avoided during?
   a. Pregnancy.
   b. Times of arthralgia.
   c. Hyperglycemic episodes.
   d. Times of fatigue.

4. Which of the following medications is contraindicated in persons receiving interleukin-2 (IL-2)?
   a. Aspirin.
   b. Acetaminophen.
   c. Antihypertensives.
   d. Steroids.

5. Biologic agents should *not* be shaken during reconstitution because this action:
   a. Increases drug side effects.
   b. Denatures biologic protein.
   c. Causes coagulation and thickening.
   d. Makes the vial explode.

6. What pattern in client body temperature will be seen in sepsis?
   a. Temperature spikes.
   b. Temperatures less than normal.
   c. Temperature is not an indicator for sepsis.
   d. Continuous low-grade fever.

7. The most common route for administration of biologic agents is:
   a. Subcutaneous.
   b. Intramuscular.
   c. Intrathecal.
   d. Intraperitoneal.

8. Your patient has received interleukin-2 treatment and has capillary leak syndrome. The signs of capillary leak syndrome are:
   a. Edema and hypotension.
   b. Increased urinary output and hyponatremia.
   c. Hypertension and dysrhythmias.
   d. Arthralgias and headache.

9. Chronic side effects of biotherapy include:
   a. Dysrhythmias and headaches.
   b. Fatigue and anorexia.
   c. Thrombocytopenia and diarrhea.
   d. Edema and decreased libido.

10. Which biologics are known for their potential to induce allergic reactions?
    a. Hematopoietic growth factors.
    b. Immunomodulators.
    c. Monoclonal antibodies.
    d. Retinoids.

*11. Which of the following side effects from use of alpha-interferon may necessitate discontinuation of the drug?
    a. Fatigue.
    b. Fever.
    c. Orthostatic hypotension.
    d. Neurotoxicity.

* Reflects advanced oncology nursing content

ANSWERS

1. **(a)**   Hematopoietic growth factors are biologic response modifiers that decrease neutropenia, anemia, and thrombocytopenia.

2. **(b)**   The generic term for protein molecules is cytokines, which include interferons, interleukins, hematopoietic growth factors, and tumor necrosis factor.

3. **(a)**   The use of retinoids should be avoided during pregnancy.

4. **(d)**   Steroid use is contraindicated in persons receiving interleukin-2.

5. **(b)**   Biologic agents should not be shaken because it denatures the protein, rendering it less effective.

6. **(a)**   Sepsis causes spikes to occur in temperature patterns.

7. **(a)**   The most common route of administration for biologic agents is subcutaneous.

8. **(a)**   Signs of capillary leak syndrome from biologics, interleukin-2, and high-dose sargramostim include decreased output, edema, hypotension, and weight gain.

9. **(b)**   Anorexia, fatigue, and personality or mental changes are chronic side effects of biotherapy.

10. **(c)**   Monoclonal antibodies have great potential to induce allergic reactions, and emergency medications, such as epinephrine, diphenhydramine, and methylprednisolone, should be kept nearby.

*11. **(d)**   Neurotoxicity may necessitate discontinuation of alpha-interferon.

* Reflects advanced oncology nursing content

CHAPTER 37

Nursing Implications of Antineoplastic Therapy

QUESTIONS

1. In which part of the cell cycle do prophase, metaphase, anaphase, and telophase occur?
   a. G_0 or resting phase.
   b. G_1 or interphase.
   c. S or synthesis.
   d. M or mitosis.

2. Which types of cancer are more sensitive to antineoplastic therapy?
   a. Those with a small tumor burden.
   b. Those with a low growth fraction.
   c. Those with a long cell cycle time.
   d. Those with cells in a G_0 phase.

3. What is the antidote for high-dose methotrexate chemotherapy?
   a. Cyclophosphamide (Cytoxan).
   b. Leucovorin.
   c. Ifosfamide.
   d. Goserelin (Zoladex).

4. Which of the following is a TRUE statement about cell cycle–specific chemotherapeutic agents?
   a. Major cytotoxic effects are exerted on cells in any phase.
   b. Agents are most effective when administered by bolus.
   c. They cost less than $10 per dose.
   d. Agents are most effective if administered in divided doses.

5. Which of the classifications of chemotherapeutic agents is cell cycle–nonspecific?
   a. Antimetabolites.
   b. Antitumor antibiotics.
   c. Plant alkaloids.
   d. Alkylating agents.

6. Which of the following chemotherapy agents is a plant alkaloid?
   a. Paclitaxel (Taxol).
   b. Cisplatin (Platinol).
   c. 5-Fluorouracil (5-FU).
   d. Methotrexate.

7. What is the name given to the classification of agents that protect against specific toxic effects of chemotherapy?
   a. Dose-limiting agents.
   b. Serotonin inhibitor agents.
   c. Topoisomerage inhibitors.
   d. Chemoprotective agents.

8. Chemotherapy drug dosages are determined by:
   a. Height only.
   b. Weight only.
   c. Body surface area.
   d. Route of administration.

9. If an extravasation of chemotherapy occurs, your first intervention should be:
   a. Call the oncologist.
   b. Remove the needle.
   c. Elevate the affected extremity.
   d. Discontinue or stop the infusion.

10. How often should intravenous patency be assessed during IV push chemotherapy?
    a. Every 0.5 mL.
    b. Every 2 to 3 mL.
    c. Every 5 mL.
    d. Every 8 to 10 mL.

11. The major toxicity associated with receiving 5-fluorouracil (5-FU) chemotherapy is:
    a. Neurotoxicity.
    b. Hemorrhagic cystitis.
    c. Cardiotoxicity.
    d. Photosensitivity.

12. The local antidote of choice if vincristine (Oncovin) extravasates is:
    a. Hyaluronidase.
    b. Sodium thiosulfate.
    c. Hydrocortisone.
    d. Diphenhydramine (Benadryl).

13. Pulmonary side effects of chemotherapy include:
    a. Phlebitis.
    b. Mucositis.
    c. Thrombocytopenia.
    d. Fibrosis.

14. Which type of cancer can be cured by single chemotherapeutic modality treatment?
    a. Pancreatic.
    b. Testicular.
    c. Breast.
    d. Liver.

15. The primary purpose of regional chemotherapy as a method of delivery is to:
    a. Enhance palliation.
    b. Increase tumor cell burden.
    c. Deliver higher doses of chemotherapy to a specific site.
    d. Act as adjuvant therapy for hormone receptor tumors.

*16. You should warm the chemotherapy solution to body temperature before administration by what route?
    a. Intrathecal.
    b. Intraarterial.
    c. Intraperitoneal.
    d. Intravesicular.

* Reflects advanced oncology nursing content

*17. Your client is having his sixth chemotherapy treatment with etoposide (VePesid), cisplatin, cyclophosphamide (Cytoxan), and doxorubicin (Adriamycin). Prior to the completion of his treatment, you note that his blood pressure is 174/98 and he is short of breath and edematous 1+. These are signs of what toxicity?
    a. Neurotoxicity.
    b. Congestive heart failure.
    c. Pulmonary fibrosis.
    d. Angioedema from anaphylaxis.

ANSWERS

1. **(d)** Cellular division occurs in prophase, metaphase, anaphase, and telophase, which are parts of mitosis.

2. **(a)** Cancers that are most sensitive to antineoplastic therapy include those with a short cell cycle, high growth fraction, and small tumor burden.

3. **(b)** Leucovorin is the antidote for high-dose methotrexate.

4. **(d)** Cell cycle–specific chemotherapy agents are most effective when administered in divided doses and are not active against cells in the G_0 or resting phase.

5. **(d)** Alkylating agents and nitrosoureas are cell cycle–nonspecific chemotherapy agents.

6. **(a)** Paclitaxel (Taxol) is a plant alkaloid.

7. **(d)** Chemoprotective agents are medications that protect against specific toxic effects of chemotherapy. Examples include dexrazoxane (Zinecard) against doxorubicin cardioxicity and amifostine (Ethyol) against cisplatin-induced myelosuppression and peripheral nervous system toxicity.

8. **(c)** Chemotherapy drug dosages are determined by body surface area, which requires measurements of height and weight.

9. **(d)** The first intervention for chemotherapeutic extravasation is to discontinue or stop the infusion.

10. **(b)** Intravenous push chemotherapy should be assessed every 2 to 3 mL for adequate intravenous patency.

11. **(d)** Photosensitivity is the major toxicity associated with administration of 5-fluorouracil (5-FU).

12. **(a)** Hyaluronidase is the local antidote to treat vincristine (Oncovin) extravasation.

13. **(d)** Edema, fibrosis, and pneumonitis are potential pulmonary side effects from chemotherapy.

14. **(b)** A single treatment modality can cure Burkitt's lymphoma, gestational trophoblastic tumors, Ewing's sarcoma, Hodgkin's disease, and testicular carcinoma.

15. **(c)** Regional chemotherapy, such as that used in liver and brain cancer, delivers higher doses of chemotherapy to specific tumor sites while reducing systematic toxicities.

*16. **(c)** Chemotherapy solutions should be warmed to body temperature before intraperitoneal administration.

*17. **(b)** Congestive heart failure is a cardiotoxic effect of doxorubicin (Adriamycin) as evidenced by edema, hypertension, and shortness of breath.

---

* Reflects advanced oncology nursing content

Principles of Preparation, Administration, and Disposal of Antineoplastic Agents

QUESTIONS

1. Short-term exposure to antineoplastic agents causes what integumentary system effect to personnel?
   a. Systemic lupus erythematosus.
   b. Dermatitis.
   c. Psoriasis.
   d. Alopecia.

2. Long-term effects to personnel after exposure to antineoplastic agents include:
   a. Thrombocytopenia.
   b. Neutropenia.
   c. Increased risk of cancer.
   d. Increased risk of pemphigus vulgaris.

3. Preparation of antineoplastic agents should occur in what type of environment?
   a. Within the nurses' station.
   b. Outside of the institution at a special antineoplastic agency.
   c. In a laminar air-flow hood.
   d. In a well-lighted room with a fan.

4. Which of the following is NOT required protective clothing when preparing antineoplastic agents?
   a. Disposable long-sleeved gown.
   b. Disposable latex gloves.
   c. Shoe covers.
   d. Plastic face shield.

5. All waste containers for antineoplastic agents must be labeled with the words:
   a. Antineoplastic refuse.
   b. Biologic and radiation contaminants.
   c. Danger: Poison containers.
   d. Caution: Chemotherapy.

*6. A nurse walks into a room where she discovers a bag of 5-fluorouracil (about 200 mL) has just leaked all over the floor. She comes out of the room yelling, "My eyes are burning." Your first response is to:
   a. Get the nurse into a shower.
   b. Complete an incident report.
   c. Flush the nurse's eyes with isotonic eyewash.
   d. Flush the nurse's eyes with 10% peroxide and water solution.

* Reflects advanced oncology nursing content

ANSWERS

1. **(b)** Dermatitis and hyperpigmentation of the skin are short-term effects of antineoplastic exposure.

2. **(c)** Alopecia, chromosome abnormalities, and increased risk of cancers are long-term effects from antineoplastic exposure.

3. **(c)** Antineoplastic agents need to be prepared in a class II, type B biologic safety cabinet with a vertical laminar air-flow hood.

4. **(c)** Shoe covers are not used in preparing antineoplastic agents. What are used are face shields or goggles, long-sleeved gowns with elastic cuffs, and latex gloves.

5. **(d)** Waste containers as well as all laboratory specimens must be labeled with the words "Caution: Chemotherapy."

*6. **(c)** Contact of chemotherapy agents to the eyes requires immediate flushing of the eyes with water or isotonic eyewash for at least 5 minutes, while holding the eyelid open.

* Reflects advanced oncology nursing content

39

Nursing Implications of Bone Marrow and Stem Cell Transplantation

QUESTIONS

1. A bone marrow transplant from a donor is call a(n):
   a. Autograph.
   b. Allograft.
   c. Identical match graft.
   d. Synergistic graft.

2. The best situation for HLA-matched donor marrow is when:
   a. Six out of six antigens match.
   b. Four out of four antigens match.
   c. Three out of three antigens match.
   d. Two out of two antigens match.

3. Autologous marrow transplants are not feasible in persons with what type of disease?
   a. Leukemia.
   b. Aplastic anemia.
   c. Breast cancer.
   d. Non-Hodgkin's lymphoma.

4. High-dose chemotherapy or total body radiation are used during what phase of the transplant process?
   a. Admission.
   b. Conditioning.
   c. Bone marrow transplant.
   d. Engraftment.

5. Clients are usually treated with a bone marrow transplant when they are:
   a. In partial remission.
   b. In complete remission.
   c. Full of cancer cells.
   d. Having central nervous system metastasis.

6. Which diagnostic procedure determines whether a client is in remission or has malignant cells present?
   a. Lumbar puncture.
   b. Computed tomography (CT) scan.
   c. Bone marrow biopsy.
   d. Serum antigen study.

7. Bone marrow is harvested using:
   a. Oral diazepam (Valium).
   b. Intravenous morphine.
   c. Oral diphenhydramine (Benadryl) plus intravenous meperidine hydrochloride (Demerol).
   d. Anesthesia.

8. After bone marrow is harvested, it is filtered. The purpose of filtering harvested bone marrow is to remove:
   a. T-cells.
   b. Fat.
   c. Hepatitis antigens.
   d. Human immunodeficiency virus (HIV).

9. Prepared marrow is infused by what route during a bone marrow transplant?
    a. Intrathecally.
    b. Intravenously.
    c. Orally.
    d. Intraarterially.

10. Critical immune system laboratory data includes all of the following for bone marrow transplant clients EXCEPT:
    a. Antinuclear antibody (ANA) titer.
    b. Cytomegalovirus (CMV) antibody titer.
    c. Epstein-Barr virus antibody titer.
    d. Herpes virus antibody titer.

11. Evaluation of the cardiovascular system is done in a person preparing for a bone marrow transplant. Which test is critical in determining cardiac output?
    a. Chest x-ray.
    b. Electrocardiogram.
    c. Cardiac ejection fraction.
    d. Arterial blood gas.

12. In reference to a client who has had an allogeneic bone marrow transplant, you hear during conference that there is evidence that "their T-lymphocytes are reacting against their tissues." This means that the client has what transplant-associated complication?
    a. Interstitial pneumonitis.
    b. Congestive heart failure (CHF).
    c. Graft-versus-host disease (GVHD).
    d. Central nervous system (CNS) metastasis.

13. What health professional should you consult to develop a plan for diversional activities for a person undergoing isolation because of bone marrow transplant?
    a. Physical therapist.
    b. Occupational therapist.
    c. Cardiac rehabilitation nurse.
    d. Dietitian.

14. The primary intervention to teach the client and family to decrease the risk of endogenous infections in a client undergoing a bone marrow transplant is:
    a. Routine oral care.
    b. Daily skin care.
    c. Visitor restriction.
    d. Meticulous handwashing.

15. When should you expect a varicella zoster virus infection to occur in a bone marrow transplant recipient?
    a. 1 week after transplant.
    b. 1 month after transplant.
    c. 2 months after transplant.
    d. 4 or more months after transplant.

16. Which of the following would be appropriate prophylactic antifungal therapy for a person after bone marrow transplant?
    a. Nystatin.
    b. Trimethoprim-sulfamethoxazole (Septra/Bactrim).
    c. Acyclovir.
    d. Pentamidine.

17. Which of the following interventions is appropriate for corneal irritation (keratitis)?
    a. Provide sunglasses.
    b. Administer mesna as prescribed.
    c. Perform routine cultures for bacteria, fungi, and viruses.
    d. Administer intravenous immunoglobins as prescribed.

18. To prevent hemorrhagic cystitis from high-dose cyclophosphamide, bladder irrigation should be implemented:
    a. Once a day.
    b. Four times a day.
    c. Every 8 hours.
    d. Continuously.

19. Your client has had a bone marrow transplant, and you are to assess for early signs of graft-versus-host disease. What body organ would be your primary area for assessment?
    a. Lungs.
    b. Lymph nodes.
    c. Skin.
    d. Spleen.

*20. Your client has had a bone marrow transplant (BMT) and complains of right upper quadrant abdominal pain along with an 8-pound weight gain in the last 24 hours. You note an elevated serum bilirubin level and some changes in mental status. What complication from BMT are you most concerned about?
    a. Graft-versus-host disease (GVHD).
    b. Interstitial pneumonitis.
    c. Cytomegalovirus infection.
    d. Hepatic venoocclusive disease.

*21. You notice that before conditioning for bone marrow transplant, the physician orders the following blood work: lactic acid dehydrogenase (LDH) and bilirubin levels. What body system is the physician assessing?
    a. Renal.
    b. Hepatic.
    c. Immune.
    d. Cardiovascular.

---

* Reflects advanced oncology nursing content

ANSWERS

1. **(b)** An allograft is a bone marrow transplant from a donor. If the donor is an identical monozygotic twin, it is called a syngeneic transplant.

2. **(a)** The best HLA-matched donor for a transplant is when six out of six antigens match.

3. **(b)** Autologous transplants are not feasible in persons with inborn bone marrow deficiency or dysfunctional bone marrow, as found in aplastic anemia.

4. **(b)** Conditioning is the phase of the transplant process in which high-dose chemotherapy or total body irradiation (TBI) are used.

5. **(b)** Clients are treated with a bone marrow transplant when they are in complete remission, because their disease is chemoresponsive at that point.

6. **(c)** A bone marrow biopsy is the diagnostic procedure done to determine if the client is in remission or still has malignant cells.

7. **(d)** Bone marrow is harvested using general or required anesthesia.

8. **(b)** Bone marrow, once harvested, is filtered to remove fat and bone particles.

9. **(b)** During a transplant, bone marrow is infused intravenously through a central venous catheter.

10. **(a)** Antibody titers for BMT clients include: CMV, Epstein-Barr, hepatitis B surface antigen, herpes virus, Ig levels, and HIV.

11. **(c)** Cardiac ejection fraction is crucial before BMT to determine the heart's ability to pump, hence the cardiac output.

12. **(c)** Graft-versus-host disease is when T-lymphocytes react against the BMT recipient's tissues. It occurs in 30% to 60% of allogeneic transplants, and there is an increased risk if six out of six HLA antigen matches are not accomplished.

13. **(b)** An occupational therapist is the person to consult to develop a plan for diversional activities during isolation of a BMT patient.

14. **(d)** It is of primary importance to teach clients and family meticulous handwashing so that endogenous infections can be avoided.

15. **(d)** Varicella zoster virus infections occur anytime after 4 months after bone marrow transplant, if they occur at all.

16. **(a)** Prophylactic antifungal therapy after BMT may include the use of clotrimazole, fluconazole, itraconazole, or nystatin.

17. **(a)** Interventions for keratitis include avoiding eye rubbing, wearing sunglasses, darkening the room, and administering artificial tears or steroid eyedrops as prescribed.

18. **(d)** Continuous bladder irrigation (CBI) is used to prevent hemorrhagic cystitis from occurring in persons treated with high-dose cyclophosphamide.

19. **(c)**   Early signs of graft-versus-host disease (GVHD) after BMT include erythema or rash on the palms of the hands and/or soles of the feet.

*20. **(d)**   Signs of hepatic venoocclusive disease after BMT include right upper quadrant abdominal pain, increased levels of serum bilirubin, weight gain of more than 5 pounds in 24 hours, change in mental status, and increased abdominal girth.

*21. **(b)**   The hepatic system is evaluated by laboratory tests for lactic acid dehydrogenase (LDH) and bilirubin levels.

---

* Reflects advanced oncology nursing content

HEALTH
PROMOTION

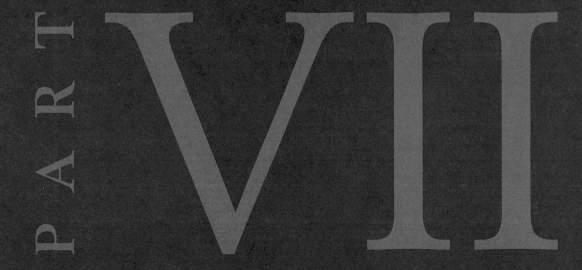

PART VII

40

Prevention of Cancer

QUESTIONS

1. Which of the following is an example of synergistic exposures to carcinogens?
    a. Radon and cotton.
    b. Weed pollen and asbestos.
    c. Alcohol and tobacco.
    d. Coal dust and microwaves.

2. Tobacco smoking is associated with an increased frequency of lung cancer and death. Tobacco smoking is a(n):
    a. Risk factor.
    b. Relative risk.
    c. Attributable risk.
    d. Promotional proto-oncogene.

3. What type of diet is an etiologic factor associated with the development of breast cancer?
    a. High-fiber.
    b. High-fat.
    c. Low-protein.
    d. Low-carbohydrate.

4. Which male has the highest relative risk of prostate cancer?
    a. Mother had breast cancer.
    b. Father and brother had prostate cancer.
    c. Brother and grandfather had prostate cancer.
    d. Mother had ovarian cancer and brother had prostate cancer.

5. An etiologic factor associated with bladder cancer is:
    a. Asbestos exposure.
    b. Low-fiber diet.
    c. Infertility.
    d. Cigarette smoking.

6. Which infectious organism increases the risk of developing gastric cancer?
    a. *Staphylococcus epidermis.*
    b. *Staphylococcus aureus.*
    c. *Helicobacter pylori.*
    d. *Escherichia coli.*

7. Living in which one of the following countries would increase a person's chance of developing malignant melanoma?
    a. South Korea.
    b. Sweden.
    c. Kenya.
    d. Spain.

8. The single most important occupational carcinogen associated with lung cancer is:
    a. Coal tar.
    b. Asbestos.
    c. Selenium.
    d. Benzene.

9. What type of energy contributes largely to the development of skin cancers?
   a. Electromagnetic fields.
   b. Ultraviolet light.
   c. Microwave energy.
   d. Cellular telephone energy.

10. Which of the following questions represents an attempt to understand the concept of perceived susceptibility to cancer?
    a. How serious do you feel cancer is?
    b. What problems do you think you will have in trying to decrease your intake of fats?
    c. Do you think you can decrease your risk for cancer if you do not smoke?
    d. How likely is it that you will develop cancer?

11. Which of the following is a strength of implementing a comprehensive cancer risk survey?
    a. Potential for aggregate data analysis.
    b. Reports based on literacy.
    c. Confidentiality not required.
    d. Reliability and validity are extremely high.

12. To best increase the chances of quitting cigarette smoking successfully, which of the following interventions should the client follow?
    a. It is all right to take a puff or two at times but never more than that.
    b. It is all right to drink alcohol, as long as it is moderate.
    c. Live in a household of total nonsmokers.
    d. Set a quit date within the next 6 months.

13. Your advice to your client regarding cancer prevention is to "drink alcohol in moderation." This means:
    a. No more than one drink of alcohol per day.
    b. One or two drinks per week.
    c. One drink per month.
    d. One drink per year.

*14. Your client is a 45-year-old construction worker who has had two basal cell carcinomas removed from his face within the last 18 months. He is married, monogamous, has four children, and lives in Texas. Your best advice to prevent further basal cell carcinomas is to:
    a. Move to Alaska.
    b. Apply sun protection factor of at least 15 every 2 to 3 hours.
    c. Wear dark-colored long-sleeve shirt whenever working.
    d. Avoid working after 12:00 noon.

*15. Your client is an employed, lower middle class woman who is illiterate, lives in a townhouse, which she owns, and whose diet is, in general, adequate. You will try to educate her regarding consistent screening behaviors associated with cancer. This client would best be educated by:
    a. Reminder card with date, time, and place of screening.
    b. Brochures on the importance of cancer screening.
    c. A flyer sent to her work location regarding the next available screening.
    d. A phone call at home to discuss cancer screening.

* Reflects advanced oncology nursing content

Answers

1. **(c)**   Synergistic exposures to carcinogens include alcohol and tobacco as well as asbestos and tobacco.

2. **(a)**   A risk factor is an element associated with the statistical increase in disease frequency, disability, or death.

3. **(b)**   A high-fat diet, in which more than 38% of calories come from fat, is an etiologic factor in the development of breast cancer.

4. **(b)**   Relative risk for prostate cancer is greatest when a client's father and brother had prostate cancer.

5. **(d)**   Cigarette smoking, radiation exposure, and phenacetin-containing analgesics are some factors associated with the development of bladder cancer.

6. **(c)**   *Helicobacter pylori*, along with a diet high in salted foods, nitrates, smoked meats, and pickled vegetables increases the risk of developing gastric cancer.

7. **(c)**   Living near the equator increases the risk of developing malignant melanoma. Kenya, in Africa, is very near the equator.

8. **(b)**   Asbestos along with radon are known occupational carcinogens associated with lung cancer.

9. **(b)**   Ultraviolet light is the main energy source that contributes to about 90% of all skin cancers.

10. **(d)**   Perceived susceptibility to cancer is understood by asking people about their likelihood of developing cancer.

11. **(a)**   A comprehensive cancer risk survey has the strength of using aggregate data for analysis and the weakness of self-reports based on unassessed literacy, reliability, and validity and the fact that confidentiality must be protected.

12. **(c)**   To quit cigarette smoking successfully a person must not drink alcohol, totally abstain from smoking, and live in a smoke-free household.

13. **(b)**   Moderate alcohol consumption means one or two drinks per week and is proper advice for cancer prevention.

*14. **(b)**   Avoiding sun exposure to prevent skin cancer includes avoiding tanning facilities, wearing long-sleeved shirts and wide-brim hats, and using sunscreen with an SPF of at least 15 every 2 to 3 hours.

*15. **(d)**   Illiteracy can be a barrier to client education, so alternate forms of communication, besides the written word, need to be used.

---

* Reflects advanced oncology nursing content

Screening and Early Detection of Cancer

QUESTIONS

1. The best realistic treatment strategy to prevent cancer in asymptomatic persons is:
   a. Screening.
   b. Surveillance.
   c. A complete physical examination yearly for all persons.
   d. Low-dose total body irradiation for those at high risk for cancer(s).

2. In 1996 in the United States, 50,000 women died from breast cancer. This is an epidemiologic example of:
   a. Prevalence.
   b. Incidence.
   c. Case-fatality.
   d. Mortality.

3. When issuing a screening test for cancer, you need to make sure that the test result will be positive if the cancer being investigated is present. This is known as test:
   a. Prediction value.
   b. Specificity.
   c. Utility.
   d. Sensitivity.

4. Screening an at-risk population for breast cancer by assessing for the BRCA-1 gene is an example of what type of screening?
   a. Mass.
   b. Selective or prescriptive.
   c. Multiple.
   d. Multiphasic.

5. Your asymptomatic patient is a 58-year-old man to whom you will need to make recommendations for early detection of cancer. Which one of the following tests would you recommend every 3 to 5 years, according to the American Cancer Society's recommendations?
   a. Digital rectal exam.
   b. Prostate exam.
   c. Fecal occult blood test.
   d. Sigmoidoscopy.

6. Cancers that are diagnosed in late stages usually show what change in client body weight?
   a. Gain in weight.
   b. Loss in weight.
   c. Neither gain nor loss.
   d. Gain from fluid buildup only.

7. Cancer-directed physical examination of the male genitalia includes:
   a. Inspection only.
   b. Palpation only.
   c. Inspection and palpation.
   d. Inspection, palpation, and percussion.

8. Which of the following tests is an endoscopic screening test for cancer?
   a. Fetal occult blood.
   b. Mammography.
   c. Pap smear.
   d. Sigmoidoscopy.

9. Which of the following serum tumor markers would most likely be elevated in a person with a hydatidiform mole?
   a. Human chorionic gonadotropin (hCG).
   b. Alkaline phosphatase.
   c. Prostate-specific antigen (PSA).
   d. Carcinoembryonic antigen (CEA).

10. Which of the following hormonal assays requires a urine sample?
    a. Androstenedione.
    b. Testosterone.
    c. 17-Ketosteroids.
    d. Parathyroid hormone.

11. What serum proteins are significant in the diagnosis of the malignancy multiple myeloma?
    a. Kupffer cells.
    b. Alpha-fetoproteins (AFPs).
    c. Immunoglobulins.
    d. Neutrophils.

12. The Seven Warning Signs of Cancer are a mnemonic for the word CAUTION. What does the "C" stand for?
    a. Consistency of wart or mole.
    b. Change in bowel or bladder habits.
    c. Cough or nagging hoarseness.
    d. Consistent bleeding or discharge.

13. How often should testicular self-examination be done?
    a. After each shower.
    b. Weekly.
    c. Monthly.
    d. Biannually.

14. To accomplish a proper self-examination of the skin what equipment is needed?
    a. A handheld mirror only.
    b. A full-length mirror only.
    c. A full-length mirror and a handheld mirror.
    d. No equipment is needed except good eyesight.

15. What serum hormonal assay is elevated in gonadotropin-producing extragonadal tumors?
    a. Calcitonin.
    b. Adrenocorticotrophic hormone (ACTH).
    c. Growth hormone (hGH).
    d. Testosterone.

16. Which of the following results of the serum tumor marker prostate-specific antigen (PSA) indicates an increase in size of the prostate, whether benign or malignant?
    a. 0.0 ng/mL.
    b. 0.5 ng/mL.
    c. 2.2 ng/mL.
    d. 5.2 ng/mL.

17. Which of the following are high-risk groups to target for cancer screening?
    a. Upper middle class.
    b. Persons with an intelligent quotient (IQ) less than 2000.
    c. Socioeconomically disadvantaged.
    d. Persons between ages 40 and 60 years old.

*18. Your client has an elevated level of CA-125 serum antigen, but there is no evidence of return of her ovarian cancer. What organ would you assess next for cancer that may also elevate CA-125 levels?
    a. Pancreas.
    b. Brain.
    c. Skin.
    d. Liver.

*19. What type of research trial controls for lead-time bias, length bias, and selection bias?
    a. Case studies.
    b. Randomized trial.
    c. Nonrandomized trial with 5-year follow-up.
    d. Controlled, homogeneous, nonrandomized trial.

* Reflects advanced oncology nursing content

ANSWERS

1. **(a)** Screening is the best strategy to prevent cancer in asymptomatic people.

2. **(d)** Mortality is an epidemiologic statistic for the number of deaths in a population over a specific period of time.

3. **(d)** Test sensitivity refers to the probability that a test result will be positive if the disease is present. If the probability is negative, then the term specificity applies.

4. **(b)** Selective or prescriptive screening is assessing high-risk populations for a specific condition, such as the BRCA-1 gene for breast cancer.

5. **(d)** Men over 55 years of age who are asymptomatic should have a sigmoidoscopy every 3 to 5 years and a yearly prostate exam, digital rectal exam, and fetal occult blood test.

6. **(b)** Persons with cancers diagnosed in late stages usually show a loss of weight.

7. **(c)** Cancer-directed physical exam of the male genitalia includes inspection and palpation.

8. **(d)** A sigmoidoscopy is an endoscopic screening test for colon cancer.

9. **(a)** hCG serum tumor marker is increased in choriocarcinoma, hydatidiform mole, and testicular teratoma.

10. **(c)** A 24-hour urine sample is required to test for 17-ketosteroids.

11. **(c)** Immunoglobulins are serum proteins produced by lymphocytes and plasma cells, which, when fractionated by electrophoresis, are diagnostic of multiple myeloma.

12. **(b)** The "C" in the Seven Warning Signs of Cancer stands for change in bowel or bladder habits.

13. **(c)** Testicular self-examination should be done monthly, after a warm bath or shower.

14. **(c)** To do a proper skin examination a full-length and handheld mirror are required.

15. **(d)** Serum testosterone levels are elevated in gonadotropin-producing extragonadal tumors.

16. **(d)** A PSA of more than 4.0 ng/mL indicates an enlarged prostate, whether benign or malignant.

17. **(c)** Target populations for cancer screening include the elderly and socioeconomically disadvantaged.

*18. **(d)** CA-125 levels can be increased with liver disease as well as ovarian cancer, breast cancer, gastrointestinal cancers, and main pulmonary cancers.

*19. **(b)** Randomized trials control for screening biases, namely lead-time bias, selection bias, and length bias.

---

* Reflects advanced oncology nursing content

PROFESSIONAL PERFORMANCE

PART VIII

42

Application of the Standards of Practice and Education

QUESTIONS

1. The component of a practice standard that explains the reason for the standard is called the:
   a. Rationale.
   b. Measurement criteria.
   c. Indicator.
   d. Compliance statement.

2. Standards of care for the professional oncology nurse include diagnosis. Diagnosis is demonstrated after:
   a. Evaluation.
   b. Planning.
   c. Implementation.
   d. Assessment.

3. Your assessment of a client from a rural town indicates that to control her ear pain she pours warm wax from a candle into her ear about four times a day. The use of this method would be recorded under what problem area?
   a. Nutrition.
   b. Comfort.
   c. Coping.
   d. Protective mechanisms.

4. The effect of alopecia on body image should be recorded under what problem area?
   a. Mobility.
   b. Protective mechanism.
   c. Circulation.
   d. Sexuality.

5. Standards of care in oncology nursing indicate that the most important person to participate in care is the:
   a. Client.
   b. Nurse.
   c. Physician.
   d. Significant other.

6. When an oncology nurse contributes to the science of nursing practice, he or she does so through what standard of professional performance?
   a. Performance appraisal.
   b. Education.
   c. Research.
   d. Resource utilization.

7. As an oncology nurse, you are ready to discharge a client and note that she is concerned about the cost of her multiple prescriptions. You solve the concern using what standard of professional performance?
   a. Ethics.
   b. Resource utilization.
   c. Education.
   d. Performance appraisal.

8. You have just taught a fellow staff nurse the side effects associated with a new medication that will begin to be used on your nursing unit tomorrow. Your contribution to your peer's professional development falls under what standard of professional performance?
   a. Quality of care.
   b. Ethics.
   c. Resource utilization.
   d. Collegiality.

9. A care plan for a person experiencing impaired skin integrity related to radiation therapy would include the wearing of clothes made out of what material?
   a. Wool.
   b. Leather.
   c. Burlap twine.
   d. Cotton.

10. Which domain of learning includes attitudes and values?
    a. Affective.
    b. Cognitive.
    c. Psychomotor.
    d. Environmental.

11. Your client demonstrates the proper physical skills for flushing his or her venous access device. What domain of learning does this represent?
    a. Affective.
    b. Cognitive.
    c. Psychomotor.
    d. Environmental.

12. Before developing a teaching plan for a client, what is the primary area that a nurse needs to assess?
    a. Available resources.
    b. Standards of care at the institution or agency.
    c. Readiness of the client to learn.
    d. Significant others' goals.

13. You are to teach and set up a 7-day menu plan for your client that is high in protein. You know that as a practicing Orthodox Catholic Christian your client does not eat meat on Fridays. What practice of the client's would influence your teaching-learning process?
    a. Ethnic.
    b. Cultural.
    c. Religious.
    d. Environmental.

*14. For each professional performance standard, there should be a preestablished level of performance that must be achieved. This preestablished level is referred to as a:
    a. Threshold.
    b. Quality of life indicator.
    c. Criterion.
    d. Eigen value.

* Reflects advanced oncology nursing content

*15. As a nurse researcher, you are concerned about the effect that spiritual issues, role changes, and employment changes have on a specific group of subjects. The best instrument to use to capture the effects of these changes would be an instrument dealing with the concept of:

a. Pain.

b. Nausea and vomiting.

c. Elimination.

d. Coping.

ANSWERS

1. **(a)**   The rationale of a practice standard explains the reason for the standard.

2. **(d)**   Diagnosis is demonstrated after assessment in standards of care for the professional oncology nurse.

3. **(b)**   Methods to control pain, including cultural and folk remedies, are recorded under the area of comfort.

4. **(d)**   The effect of treatment side effects on body image are recorded under sexuality as a problem area.

5. **(a)**   The client is the most important person to participate in care, according to the standards of care in oncology nursing.

6. **(c)**   Contributing to the science of nursing practice is done through the standard of professional performance called research.

7. **(b)**   Concern over issues of cost, safety, and effectiveness fall under the standard of resource utilization under professional performance.

8. **(d)**   Collegiality is the standard of professional performance in which a nurse contributes to the professional development of colleagues, peers, and others.

9. **(d)**   Clothes made out of cotton are suggested for persons experiencing impaired skin integrity from radiation therapy because cotton is soft, decreases friction, does not irritate, and breathes.

10. **(a)**   The affective domain of learning includes attitudes and values.

11. **(c)**   The psychomotor domain of learning includes physical skills, such as flushing a venous access device.

12. **(c)**   Before developing a teaching plan, a nurse must assess the client's level of education and readiness to learn.

13. **(c)**   Religious practices, along with cultural and ethnic practices, should be investigated in relation to the teaching-learning process.

*14. **(a)**   A threshold is a preestablished level of performance that should be achieved for each professional performance standard.

*15. **(d)**   Coping deals with the effects of employment changes, role changes, and spiritual concerns.

---

* Reflects advanced oncology nursing content

43

The Education Process

QUESTIONS

1. What type of education is aimed at improving professional performance to improve client and community health?
   a. Health education.
   b. Client education.
   c. Staff education.
   d. Public education.

2. Which of the following is a theoretical principle of teaching and learning?
   a. Learning should be problem-centered, not subject-centered.
   b. Learning occurs if teaching is done.
   c. There is no need to include repetition in adult learning.
   d. A teaching plan should include practice opportunities only if the client has asked for them.

3. Which of the following physical factors is appropriate for a positive learning environment?
   a. Minimal lighting.
   b. Hard chairs with straight, upright backs.
   c. Two speakers answering different questions at the same time.
   d. Two feet of room between each person.

4. Which of the following is an emotional response that can lead to a decrease in the client's receptiveness to learning?
   a. Fear.
   b. Fatigue.
   c. Pain.
   d. Sleep deprivation.

5. Assessment of a client's socioeconomic status is part of a complete assessment of the education process. Which one of the following terms reflects socioeconomic status?
   a. Concrete thinking skills.
   b. Belief in a higher being.
   c. Lifestyle.
   d. Beliefs.

6. The steps of the educational process consist of assessment, diagnosis, planning, implementation, and:
   a. Repetition.
   b. Evaluation.
   c. Motivation.
   d. Mutual respect.

*7. The nursing diagnosis of ineffective individual coping is most notable in what phase of the cancer experience?
   a. Diagnostic.
   b. Surveillance.
   c. Prediagnostic.
   d. Bereavement.

* Reflects advanced oncology nursing content

ANSWERS

1. **(c)**   Staff education is designed to improve professional performance so the outcome can be improvement of client, family, and community health.

2. **(a)**   Theoretical principles of teaching and learning include a problem-centered approach with reinforcement and practice opportunities.

3. **(d)**   A positive learning environment includes adequate space, privacy, good lighting, comfortable seats, and few to no distractions.

4. **(a)**   Emotional responses that can affect responsiveness to learning include anxiety, anger, fear, depression, and distrust.

5. **(c)**   Examples of socioeconomic status that a nurse assesses in relation to the education process include use of leisure time, lifestyle, and work situation.

6. **(b)**   The stages of the educational process include assessment, diagnosis, planning, implementation, and evaluation.

*7. **(a)**   Ineffective individual coping is the nursing diagnosis most noted in the diagnostic phase of the cancer experience in which the focus is on workup and supporting the client in coping with the diagnosis of cancer.

* Reflects advanced oncology nursing content

CHAPTER

44

Legal Issues Influencing Cancer Nursing

QUESTIONS

1. Which professional document provides the definition and role of nursing in each state in the United States?
   a. American Nurses' Association (ANA) Standards of Practice.
   b. Oncology Nursing Society (ONS) Standards of Oncology Nursing.
   c. Nurse Practice Acts.
   d. Joint Commission on Accreditation of Healthcare Organizations (JCAHO).

2. What term of liability is defined as a deviation from a professional standard of care?
   a. Negligence.
   b. Malpractice.
   c. Breach of duty.
   d. Incomplete accountability.

3. Litigation involving the fact that the nurse did not give a client leucovorin following high-dose methotrexate involves a(n):
   a. Lack of teaching.
   b. Inadequate referral.
   c. Medication error.
   d. Insufficient discharge plan.

4. What is the name of the patient rights organization that protects the constitutional rights of United States citizens?
   a. The National Hospice Organization.
   b. American Civil Liberties Union (ACLU).
   c. Citizen Advocacy Center (CAC).
   d. National Health Law Program.

5. Which of the following terms is associated with labor relations?
   a. Staff mix.
   b. Advanced directives.
   c. Collective bargaining.
   d. Unlicensed assistive personnel (UAP).

6. The number one reported disciplinary action by state boards of nursing is:
   a. Staff tardiness.
   b. Client neglect.
   c. Stealing hospital or client possessions.
   d. Chemical dependency.

*7. An institutional policy states that if you have 10 clients, you should have a minimum of two registered nurses on duty at all times. A statute states that if you have 10 clients, you should have a minimum of three registered nurses on duty at all times. As the nurse manager, you have 10 clients and two registered nurses scheduled for duty on the 3:00 PM to 11:00 PM shift. Your knowledge of agency and institutional policies and procedures assures you that:
   a. Institutional policy overrides all other policies.
   b. Only a superior court judge can change nurse/client ratios.
   c. Statutes override institutional policies.
   d. As a member of management you can legally decide to override the statute.

---

* Reflects advanced oncology nursing content

ANSWERS

1. **(c)** The nurse practice acts of each state provide the definition and role of nursing for that state.

2. **(b)** Malpractice is defined as a deviation from a professional standard of care.

3. **(c)** Medication errors by commission or omission are areas for litigation, such as omission of leucovorin rescue following high-dose methotrexate.

4. **(b)** The American Civil Liberties Union (ACLU) is the organization that protects citizens' constitutional rights.

5. **(c)** Collective bargaining is a term associated with labor relations and is becoming more prevalent in the health care system.

6. **(d)** The number one disciplinary action by state boards of nursing is for chemical dependency, which affects about 10% of all nurses.

*7. **(c)** Statutes override regulations. Regulations override institutional policies.

---

* Reflects advanced oncology nursing content

Selected Ethical Issues in Cancer Care

QUESTIONS

1. Influencing a person to act against his or her will is the definition of what inappropriate factor regarding obtaining informed consent?
   a. Coercion.
   b. Deception.
   c. Paternalism.
   d. Captivity.

2. During the process of informed consent, you explain to the client that this research therapy "may kill all your cancer cells." This statement reflects an explanation of known:
   a. Coercion.
   b. Benefits.
   c. Alternatives.
   d. Consequences of refusing therapy.

3. During the process of informed consent, who is responsible for explaining medical treatments and procedures?
   a. Staff nurse.
   b. Nurse manager or administrator.
   c. Physician assistant.
   d. Physician.

4. A "Do Not Resuscitate" (DNR) decision means that cardiopulmonary resuscitation is not performed in the event the client's:
   a. Respirations only cease.
   b. Pulse only ceases.
   c. Either respirations or pulse ceases.
   d. Both respirations and pulse ceases.

*5. Which of the following quantitative research designs requires incomplete disclosure?
   a. Case study.
   b. Double-blind experiments.
   c. Descriptive study.
   d. Grounded theory.

* Reflects advanced oncology nursing content

ANSWERS

1. **(a)** Coercion is defined as influencing a person to act against his or her own will and is inappropriate in obtaining informed consent.

2. **(b)** Benefits of informed consent include possible positive outcomes. Other areas of explanation include risks, alternatives, and consequences of not accepting treatment.

3. **(d)** The physician is responsible for explaining medical treatments and procedures during informed consent.

4. **(d)** A DNR decision means no CPR is performed if *both* the client's respirations and pulse cease.

*5. **(b)** Double-blind experiments are quantitative research designs that require incomplete disclosure because full knowledge would affect the results of the study.

---

* Reflects advanced oncology nursing content

CHAPTER 46

Cancer Economics and Health Care Reform

QUESTIONS

1. Managed care reimbursement, in which there is a fixed amount paid per day regardless of the ancillary services provided, is the definition of:
   a. Global case rate.
   b. Discounts.
   c. Per diem.
   d. Capitation.

2. In which type of cancer environment are there unlimited referrals for health care delivery?
   a. Nonmanaged care.
   b. Health maintenance organization (HMO).
   c. Independent practice association (IPA).
   d. Preferred provider organization (PPO).

3. Which of the following statements is TRUE about end-of-life care for cancer patients?
   a. Intensive care unit (ICU) care increases life by 5 years.
   b. Most patients spend 1 to 2 years at home after discharge.
   c. The last year of life costs approximately 75% of total lifetime health care costs.
   d. Medicare has few costs associated with end-of-life care.

4. Your client is reimbursed by his or her insurance carrier for medical expenses. What type of insurance does your client have?
   a. Life insurance.
   b. Indemnity insurance.
   c. Physician hospital organization (PHO) insurance.
   d. Per case insurance.

5. What type of managed care reimbursement pays a fixed amount per stay regardless of how long you stay?
   a. Per case.
   b. Global care.
   c. Capitation.
   d. Per diem.

6. Which of the following is a technologic advance in radiation therapy?
   a. Positron emission tomography (PET).
   b. Monoclonal antibodies.
   c. Proton beam therapy.
   d. Stereotactic resonance marker therapy.

7. Health care reform that deals with placing capitations on pain and suffering and limits attorney fees is called what type of legislative reform?
   a. Provider reform.
   b. Scope of practice reform.
   c. Malpractice litigation reform.
   d. Health service planning reform.

*8. Your colleague asks you which type of health care is better, nonmanaged care or managed care. After asking your colleague several questions you learn that he or she is interested in prevention and believes all physicians are the same, but there is a preference for a primary care model. You therefore recommend:

　a. Nonmanaged care.
　b. Managed care.
　c. Neither because both are so similar.
　d. Being uninsured because the government pays the bills anyway.

ANSWERS

1. **(c)**   Per diem is reimbursement at a fixed amount per day, regardless of the ancillary services provided.

2. **(a)**   Unlimited referrals are found in nonmanaged care environments.

3. **(c)**   End-of-life care costs are high: about 75% of total lifetime health care costs.

4. **(b)**   Indemnity insurance is coverage where the client or insured is reimbursed by the insurance company.

5. **(a)**   Per case managed care reimbursement is a fixed amount per stay no matter the length of time you stay.

6. **(c)**   Managed care often challenges technologic advances and thereby refuses coverage. Advances made in radiation therapy include proton beam therapy, multileaf collimator, stereotactic radiosurgery, and conformal therapy.

7. **(c)**   Malpractice litigation reform deals with limits on attorney fees and limits on liability and capitation set for pain and suffering.

*8. **(b)**   Managed care focuses on prevention, uses only selected groups of physicians, and uses a primary care model.

---

* Reflects advanced oncology nursing content

Changes in Oncology Health Care Settings

QUESTIONS

1. A decision-making process that anticipates needs of the client and family is called:
   a. Reactive.
   b. Proactive.
   c. Ongoing.
   d. Collaborative.

2. Which member of the health care team has expertise in community support and spiritual care?
   a. Case manager.
   b. Nurse.
   c. Social worker.
   d. Priest, chaplain, minister, or rabbi.

3. Outpatient oncology settings are primarily concerned with providing care for clients requiring:
   a. Conventional chemotherapy.
   b. Phase I drug studies.
   c. High-dose investigational therapy.
   d. Critical care.

4. What would be the best care setting for a 40-year-old woman who is terminally ill and has two children aged 16 and 18 and a husband?
   a. Ambulatory care.
   b. Subacute care.
   c. Hospice care.
   d. Skilled nursing care.

5. Professional burnout of oncology nurses is related to all of the following EXCEPT:
   a. Poor pay.
   b. Staffing shortages.
   c. Frustrating family demands.
   d. Personal psychological strains.

6. What resource is not usually available to oncology nurses in the rural setting to help provide optimal cancer-related care?
   a. Professional cancer journals.
   b. Cancer textbooks.
   c. Regional or national seminars.
   d. Internet computer consultation.

7. The home care setting significantly reduces the incidence of infection in what organ?
   a. Heart.
   b. Wound.
   c. Lungs.
   d. Oral cavity.

8. What type of hospice program has no facility except an office?
   a. Community-based program.
   b. Inpatient-based program.
   c. Inpatient-based hospice team program.
   d. Freestanding hospice.

9. The primary area of nursing care emphasized in hospice care is:
   a. Dietary management.
   b. Pain control.
   c. Informed consent for clinical trials.
   d. Pulmonary hygiene.

10. When the primary caregiver needs respite time and home health care is not adequate, what is the best option for client care?
    a. Skilled nursing facility.
    b. Inpatient hospitalization.
    c. Hospice care.
    d. Personal home care.

11. When is hospice care completed?
    a. On the client's death.
    b. After bereavement follow-up.
    c. After the client's funeral.
    d. After the significant other's or spouse's death.

12. Which of the following is a high-acuity support service available through home care?
    a. Enemas.
    b. Arterial pump chemotherapy.
    c. Gastric tube feedings.
    d. Pulse oximetry.

13. In the home care setting, who has the role as first-line observer for changes in the client's health status?
    a. Physician.
    b. Home health nurse.
    c. Home care provider.
    d. Next door neighbor.

14. Which one of the following is NOT a licensed health care worker?
    a. Registered nurse (RN).
    b. Licensed vocational nurse (LVN).
    c. Licensed practical nurse (LPN).
    d. Certified nursing assistant (CNA).

15. Which of the following is TRUE about hospice care?
    a. Use of multidisciplinary teams is prohibited.
    b. Client's may NOT continue in cancer therapy.
    c. Medicare clients are NOT eligible for hospice care.
    d. Care includes around-the-clock commitment.

*16. Rehabilitation issues of speech and maintenance of optimal nutrition are associated with cancer of the:
    a. Lung.
    b. Head and neck.
    c. Breast.
    d. Bladder.

* Reflects advanced oncology nursing content

*17. A friend has just been diagnosed with stage II Hodgkin's disease. She has chosen to receive intravenous combination chemotherapy for treatment. Which of the following oncology specialists will your friend need?
   a. Surgical oncologist.
   b. Palliative care oncologist.
   c. Medical oncologist.
   d. Radiation oncologist.

ANSWERS

1. **(b)**   Proactive processes anticipate the needs of clients and family members.

2. **(d)**   A priest, chaplain, minister, or rabbi is a member of the health care team who has expertise in community support and spiritual care.

3. **(a)**   Conventional chemotherapy is primarily administered in an outpatient setting.

4. **(c)**   Hospice care is an appropriate setting for a terminally ill client.

5. **(a)**   Oncology burnout is not related to issues of pay or salary.

6. **(d)**   Internet computer consultations are not usually available to oncology nurses in rural settings.

7. **(c)**   The incidence of pulmonary infections is significantly decreased in the home care setting.

8. **(a)**   A community-based hospice has no facility, just an office, and home care is the focus.

9. **(b)**   Pain control is the primary area of nursing care in a hospice.

10. **(a)**   A skilled nursing facility is a good care option for a client when the primary caregiver needs respite time and home health care is not adequate.

11. **(b)**   Hospice care is completed after bereavement follow-up.

12. **(b)**   High-acuity support services available through home care include chemotherapy administration via arterial pump, intravenous, intrathecal, or peritoneal routes.

13. **(c)**   The home care provider is the first-line observer for changes in a client's health status in a home care setting.

14. **(d)**   A certified nursing assistant is not a licensed health care worker.

15. **(d)**   Hospice care includes a 24-hour-a-day commitment, use of multidisciplinary teams, cancer therapy may be continued, and Medicare clients are eligible since legislation in 1983 in the United States.

*16. **(b)**   Cancer of the head and neck involves rehabilitation issues of nutritional maintenance, shoulder or neck dysfunction, speech, appearance, and self-care.

*17. **(c)**   A medical oncologist is an oncology specialist who deals with persons receiving intravenous combination chemotherapy.

---

* Reflects advanced oncology nursing content

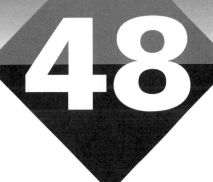

CHAPTER

48

Professional Issues
in Cancer Care

QUESTIONS

1. What characteristic of a profession means self-governing or self-regulating?
   a. Autonomy.
   b. Authority.
   c. Commitment.
   d. Competency.

2. An appropriate referral for a post-operative head and neck cancer client to regain use of an affected shoulder is a referral to:
   a. Hospice.
   b. Home care.
   c. Rehabilitation.
   d. Palliative care.

3. Which type of working relationship provides synergism of talents in a true partnership?
   a. Slave-master relationship.
   b. Detente relationship.
   c. Commonality relationship.
   d. Collaboration relationship.

4. Collaboration among medical oncology nurses, surgical oncology nurses, and radiation oncology nurses is known as collaboration among:
   a. Roles.
   b. Specialists.
   c. Subspecialists.
   d. Domains of responsibility.

5. Acute care, outpatient, home care, and hospice are words that describe:
   a. Practice settings.
   b. Roles.
   c. Subspecialties.
   d. Attitudes.

6. At what level of research preparation should a nurse be able to conduct independent research investigation?
   a. Associate degree.
   b. Baccalaureate degree.
   c. Master's degree.
   d. Doctorate degree.

7. What research studies are restricted to National Cancer Institute (NCI)–designated centers?
   a. Double-blind studies.
   b. Cooperative group studies.
   c. Phase I studies.
   d. Psychosocial studies.

8. Obtaining subjects that meet research protocol requirements is called:
   a. Client accrual.
   b. Collecting data.
   c. Identification of clinical variables.
   d. Observing client responses.

9. Which of the following would be an indication that your employer supports nursing research?
   a. Research role is included in your job description.
   b. There is no research budget.
   c. There is no nursing research committee.
   d. The director of nursing research is also the director of hospital security.

10. The purpose of what type of research is to describe relationships and cause and effect?
    a. Surveys.
    b. Phenomenologic.
    c. Qualitative.
    d. Quantitative.

11. A statement about the importance of the research study is found in what section of a research report?
    a. Research problem.
    b. Theoretical framework.
    c. Methodology.
    d. Discussion.

12. One of the funding resources for nursing research is the International Honor Society of Nursing. This organization is also known as:
    a. The American Nurses' Foundation.
    b. The National League for Nurses.
    c. Sigma Theta Tau.
    d. The National Center for Nursing Research.

13. When does stress become problematic?
    a. When it promotes growth.
    b. When one responds effectively.
    c. When coping mechanisms fail.
    d. When resources are adequate.

14. Which of the following is a characteristic within the work setting that is a stressor for the oncology nurse?
    a. Nurse is overly dedicated.
    b. Organizational change occurs in the care delivery system.
    c. Nurse is idealistic.
    d. Home conflicts.

15. What is the name of the process when professional nurses appraise the quality of care provided by fellow nurses?
    a. Licensure.
    b. Professional certification.
    c. Peer review.
    d. Accountability.

16. The purpose of certification in nursing is to:
    a. Increase the revenue of associations.
    b. Enforce the Patient Bill of Rights.
    c. Increase monetary compensation for staff nurses.
    d. Recognize expert practitioners.

17. Nurse/client ratio is an example of what type of criterion in quality improvement monitoring?
    a. Structure.
    b. Process.
    c. Outcome.
    d. Health status.

18. The nurse practice act includes conviction for a felony as grounds for disciplinary action. What is the administrative agency that implements the statutes of the nurse practice act in the United States?
    a. The Joint Commission on Accreditation of Healthcare Organizations.
    b. The American Nurses' Association.
    c. The Board of Nursing.
    d. The National Institute of Health.

19. Doing something to a person without his or her consent but for the person's own good is an example of what type of advocacy?
    a. Simplistic.
    b. Paternalistic.
    c. Consumer.
    d. Existential.

20. Which of the following is a physical response to stress?
    a. Fatigue.
    b. Irritability.
    c. Forgetfulness.
    d. Feelings of powerlessness.

21. Which of the following is an intellectual response to stress?
    a. Feelings of guilt.
    b. Lack of concentration.
    c. Whining.
    d. Neck pain.

*22. You have a staff nurse employee who is cynical and has negative feelings toward some clients and most coworkers. Your plan to help the employee should include assistance in the area of:
    a. Time management.
    b. Acknowledgment of vulnerabilities.
    c. Adopting a wellness philosophy.
    d. Attitude change.

*23. Which of the following is an example of an inferential statistic that predicts differences or relationships?
    a. Frequencies.
    b. Standard deviation.
    c. Analysis of variance.
    d. Mean.

* Reflects advanced oncology nursing content

ANSWERS

1. **(a)** Autonomy is defined as self-governing or self-regulating and is a professional characteristic.

2. **(c)** A referral to rehabilitation can help a post-operative head and neck cancer client regain shoulder movement.

3. **(d)** Collaboration is the type of working relationship that is a true partnership and provides synergism of talents.

4. **(c)** Collaboration among subspecialists includes persons in medical, surgical, radioactive, and biotherapy oncology nursing. Collaboration among specialists occurs among oncology nurses, critical care nurses, and intraoperative nurses.

5. **(a)** Practice settings in oncology are numerous. Some examples include acute care, outpatient care, home care, ambulatory care, and hospice care.

6. **(d)** Independent research investigation can be conducted by a nurse prepared at the doctorate level.

7. **(c)** Phase I studies are restricted to NCI–designated centers.

8. **(a)** Client accrual is the term used when a research nurse obtains subjects that meet research protocol requirements.

9. **(a)** Support of nursing research by an employer is positive if nursing research is included in the job description, there is a nursing research committee with a budget, and a nurse researcher is the director of nursing research.

10. **(d)** The purpose of quantitative research is to describe relationships and cause and effect.

11. **(a)** A statement about the importance of the research study is found in the section of the research report entitled "Statement of the Research Problem and Purpose."

12. **(c)** Sigma Theta Tau International Honor Society of Nursing funds nursing research as does NCNR, ANF, ONS, and AACN.

13. **(c)** Stress becomes problematic when a person cannot cope effectively, leading to compromises in client care, physical or emotional distress, and job burnout.

14. **(b)** Characteristics within the work setting that are stressors to oncology nurses include organizational changes in delivery of care, inadequate staffing, limited autonomy, limited upward mobility, inadequate support from peers, and unclear roles.

15. **(c)** Peer review is the process of nurses appraising the quality of care provided by fellow nurses.

16. **(d)** The purpose of certification in areas of nursing includes the recognition of expert practitioners and protection of the public.

17. **(a)** Nurse/client ratio is an example of a structural criterion used to describe organizational attributes in quality improvement or quality assurance.

18. (c) The Board of Nursing in each state in the United States is the administrative agency that implements the statutes of the nurse practice act.

19. (b) Paternalistic advocacy is when you do something for or to a person for his or her own good but without the person's consent.

20. (a) Fatigue, sleep disturbances, and changes in physical appearance and sexual behavior are physical responses to stress.

21. (b) Intellectual responses to stress include forgetfulness, lack of concentration, preoccupation, tardiness, and mathematical errors.

*22. (d) Employees who are cynical and display negative feelings toward clients and coworkers need help in changing their attitude.

*23. (c) Analysis of variance (ANOVA), t-test, and χ^2 (chi square) are examples of inferential statistics that predict differences and relationships.

---

* Reflects advanced oncology nursing content

Issues and Challenges in Alternative Therapies

QUESTIONS

1. Another name for conventional medicine is the term:
   a. Folk.
   b. Orthodox.
   c. Natural.
   d. Homeopathic.

2. Which of the following is an example of an alternate therapy whose aim is to reduce stress?
   a. Use of garlic-containing foods.
   b. Shark cartilage infusions.
   c. Biofeedback.
   d. Coffee enemas.

3. Alternate therapies appeal largely to:
   a. Rural patients.
   b. Poorly educated persons.
   c. Well-educated persons.
   d. People with low income.

4. The primary intervention associated with having a client informed about biomedical options and alternative therapies is:
   a. Open communication.
   b. Cultural insensitivity.
   c. Having a judgmental attitude.
   d. Quick dismissal of any talk about alternative therapies.

*5. Your client comes in for his chemotherapy treatment and states, "You know, I'm taking vitamin E, laetrile, and a natural product to boost my immune system. I sure hope it helps." Your best response to this statement is:
   a. "You're too smart to take all that junk."
   b. "Why don't you tell me more about these products."
   c. "If you take these products and the doctor finds out, I'm afraid what will happen to you."
   d. "These products are just ways to take your money."

* Reflects advanced oncology nursing content

ANSWERS

1. **(b)**   Another name used to describe conventional medicine is orthodox.

2. **(c)**   Biofeedback and yoga are alternative therapies in which the aim is to reduce stress.

3. **(c)**   Alternative therapies appeal mostly to well-educated, middle-class people who live in an urban setting.

4. **(a)**   Open communication is the primary intervention for having a client informed about biomedical options and alternative therapy options.

*5. **(b)**   When a client is involved in alternative therapies, the best approach is to maintain open lines of communication, avoid quick dismissals, and to be sensitive and nonjudgmental.

---

* Reflects advanced oncology nursing content

INDEX